MAKING
HEALTH CARE
DECISIONS

The following chapters of this book are also available in booklet format from Liguori Publications

Making Health Care Decisions:
A Catholic Guide: Introduction
Ron Hamel
ISBN 0-7648-1406-0

Making Health Care Decisions:
A Catholic Guide to End-of-Life Care
Richard C. Sparks
ISBN 0-7648-1404-4

Making Health Care Decisions:
A Catholic Guide to
Advance Health Care Directives
Mark Miller
ISBN 0-7648-1403-6

Making Health Care Decisions:
A Catholic Guide to Medically Administered
Nutrition and Hydration
Michael R. Panicola
ISBN 0-7648-1405-2

Order from www.liguori.org or call toll-free 1-800-325-9521.

MAKING HEALTH CARE DECISIONS

A Catholic Guide

EDITED BY RON HAMEL

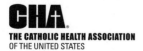

THE CATHOLIC HEALTH ASSOCIATION
OF THE UNITED STATES

Liguori
LIGUORI, MISSOURI

Imprimi Potest: Thomas D. Picton, C.Ss.R.
Provincial, Denver Province, The Redemptorists

Published by Liguori Publications, Liguori, Missouri
www.liguori.org

Library of Congress Cataloging-in-Publication Data

Hamel, Ron.
    Making health care decisions : a Catholic guide / edited by Ronald P. Hamel.—1st ed.
        p. cm.
    Includes index.
    ISBN 10: 0-7648-1402-8; ISBN 13: 978-0-7648-1402-0 (pbk.)
    1. Medical ethics—Religious aspects—Catholic Church. 2. Medical care—Religious aspects—Catholic Church. I. Hamel, Ronald P. 1946–. II. Title. [DNLM: 1. Catholicism—Popular Works. 2. Ethics, Clinical—Popular Works. 3. Patient Participation—Popular Works. 4. Religion and Medicine—Popular Works. WB 60 M235 2006]
R725.56.M27 2006
174.2—dc22   2006005384

Printed in the United States of America
10 09 08 07 06   5 4 3 2 1
First edition

Contents

Contributors

M. Therese Lysaught, PhD, is associate professor of the Department of Religious Studies at the University of Dayton.

Patricia Talone, RSM, PhD, is vice president, Mission Services, at the Catholic Health Association of the United States in St. Louis.

Ron Hamel, PhD, is Senior Director, Ethics, at the Catholic Health Association of the United States in St. Louis.

Richard C. Sparks, CSSP, PhD, is a Paulist priest and pastor of Newman Hall-Holy Spirit parish in Berkeley, California, and a frequent lecturer and writer on moral issues.

Carol Tauer, PhD, professor of Philosophy Emerita, College of St. Catherine, St. Paul and Visiting Professor, Center for Bioethics, University of Minnesota.

Mark Miller, C.Ss.R., PhD, is a Redemptorist priest, director of the Redemptorist Bioethics Consultancy, an ethicist at St. Paul's Hospital and the Saskatoon Health District, Saskatoon, Canada, and he teaches at St. Thomas More College, Saskatoon.

Michael R. Panicola, PhD, is corporate vice president of Ethics for SSM Health Care in St. Louis and adjunct professor of health care ethics, theological studies, and health management and policy at St. Louis University.

Sponsoring Organizations

Liguori Publications

The mission of Liguori Publications, a collaborative effort of Redemptorists and laity, is to spread the Gospel of Jesus Christ primarily through the print and electronic media. The founder of the Redemptorists, Alphonsus Liguori—saint and doctor of the Church—is widely regarded as one of the greatest moral theologians of all time. *Making Health Care Decisions: A Catholic Guide* advances this moral foundation and supports the healing ministry of Jesus. For more information about Liguori Publications, see www.liguori.org.

The Catholic Health Association of the United States

The Catholic Health Association of the United States (CHA USA), founded in 1915, exists to support and strengthen the Catholic health ministry—and thus the healing ministry of Jesus—in the United States, particularly in the areas of mission, ethics, and advocacy. For more information about the Catholic Health Association, see www.chausa.org.

Introduction

C onsider for a moment the many headlines that have appeared in newspapers and on the evening news during the first five years of the twenty-first century that announced some new medical breakthrough or major event with implications for health care. Advances in science, technology, and patient care provide hope for the future, but with each new move forward comes new challenges.

On April 14, 2003, for example, the completion of the human genome project was announced. All 3.1 billion base pairs of the human genome (found in the nucleus of virtually every cell in the human body) had been sequenced. The information gained from that thirteen-year endeavor will lead to further discoveries about how genes function in the body; how they interact with one another, the environment, and lifestyle choices; and how particular genes contribute to specific diseases. This and other information will increase our capacity to prevent, diagnose, and treat genetic disorders that cause untold suffering. Many scientists believe that the mapping of the human genome will eventually revolutionize medicine. With the ongoing and relatively frequent discovery of more and more genes that play a role in specific diseases, increasing numbers of genetic tests will be developed to determine the presence of mutant genes which, in turn, is likely to lead to increasing expectations that physicians will offer these tests. Already, scientists have developed tests for over one thousand disorders, including some forms of breast cancer, Alzheimer's, Parkinson's, ALS, and colon cancer.

Or think about the summer of 2001, the "summer of stem cell research." In July, the Jones Institute, a well-known fertility clinic in Virginia, announced that it had created human embryos *in vitro* as an additional source for obtaining human embryonic stem cells. That same month, Advanced Cell Technology, a biotech firm in Massachusetts, announced that it was attempting to clone human embryos for therapeutic purposes, especially for obtaining stem cells. In August, the House of Representatives passed a bill banning all human cloning, but the Democratic-led Senate tabled the companion bill. That same month, President George W. Bush announced on national television that federal funds could be used for human embryonic stem cell research only on already existing embryonic stem cell lines (because the destruction of human embryos had already occurred) to the dismay of many on both the right and the left. Finally, in November 2001, Advanced Cell Technology announced that it had successfully cloned human embryos using both somatic cell nuclear transfer and parthenogenesis (stimulating an unfertilized egg to develop), although every embryo died before stem cells could be obtained.

The issue of human embryonic stem cell research has not diminished in visibility or intensity since the summer of 2001. Many states across the nation either have considered or are considering legislation that would either prohibit or permit human cloning for research purposes, especially for obtaining stem cells. Likewise, battles are being waged in state legislatures over the use of state funds for human embryonic stem cell research. Several states—California, New Jersey, and Connecticut to date—have passed laws or initiatives to fund such research. Biotech companies continue to develop stem cell lines, destroying human embryos in the process. Stanford University announced in December 2002 its plans to pursue cloning as a source of stem cells; in April 2004, Harvard University established the Harvard Stem Cell Institute devoted to advancing the science of stem cells from the laboratory to clinical applications. In February 2004, Korean scientists claimed to have derived stem cells from cloned human embryos, though these claims have since been largely discredited.

Or recall the vehement controversy, played out on television before the entire world and in local newspapers across the country, over the withdrawal of Terri Schiavo's feeding tube. The controversy focused on whether it was morally and legally permissible to withdraw Ms. Schaivo's feeding tube (as well as the feeding tube of other patients in a persistent vegetative state) and whether her husband had the authority to do so. Fueling the controversy was a talk given by Pope John Paul II on March 20, 2004, in which he described tube feeding as an ordinary means of sustaining life and, therefore, generally morally obligatory for patients in a persistent vegetative state. These two events have left a cloud of doubt over the moral permissibility of withholding or withdrawing medically administered nutrition and hydration particularly in patients in PVS, but in other patients as well. They have also raised concerns about advance health care directives and whether it is morally permissible to stipulate in one's advance directive that one does not want to be kept alive by feeding tubes. Some state legislatures have revised their advance directive legislation to exclude the removal of feeding tubes from any patient unless that patient has expressly stipulated in written form to the contrary. Some Catholic dioceses have issued a "Catholic Living Will" which does not allow for the removal of a feeding tube.

These and numerous other developments in science, medicine, and the health care arena, in just the first five years of this century, either have touched or will impact each of us in one way or another. And such developments will continue to occur, most likely at an even faster pace and with increasing complexity. They will require real-life decisions—about one's own medical care or that of a loved one, or about state and national public policies. Decisions of this significance ought not be made lightly. They should be well informed, arrived at carefully and collaboratively, taking into account the experience and wisdom of others and the promptings of one's own informed conscience. There is much at stake in how we make these decisions—for ourselves, our families, our organizations, and the communities in which we live. At issue are how our choices impact real people and how they shape the kinds of people, families, organizations, and communities we become.

Making Health Care Decisions: A Catholic Guide

This book is intended primarily for Catholics—Catholics "in the pews" and Catholics in various types of health care institutions and organizations. It is meant to provide some guidance through the complexities of several areas that are prominent in the health care arena today. Any number of issues could have been chosen for this volume. Those that have been chosen were selected precisely because they are likely to directly affect many people and about which people must make decisions—stem cells, genetic testing, organ transplantation, end-of-life issues, advance health care directives, and medically administered nutrition and hydration.

Each of these topics is discussed in light of the moral guidance provided by the Church. Regarding some issues, the Church has a very clear position. Human embryonic stem cell research, for example, is condemned by the Church because it involves the destruction of human embryos. With regard to other issues, however, there is no specific official teaching. In these instances, the Church may offer moral principles to guide the making of moral decisions or the guidance to be derived from fundamental values drawn from the Hebrew and Christian scriptures, the Catholic theological and moral tradition, and Catholic social teaching, such as respect for human dignity, concern for the poor and vulnerable, and contributing to the common good.

When confronting moral issues, each one of us must ultimately follow the dictates of our conscience in deciding what to do. The Catholic tradition has been clear about this through the centuries as eloquently synthesized in the Second Vatican Council's *Pastoral Constitution on the Church in the Modern World* (par. 16).

> In the depths of our conscience, we detect a law which we do not impose upon ourselves, but which holds us to obedience. Always summoning us to love good and avoid evil, the voice of conscience when necessary speaks to our hearts: do this, shun that. For we have in our hearts a law written by God; to obey it is the very dignity of the human person; according to it we will be judged. Conscience is the most secret core and sanctuary of a person. There we are alone with God, whose voice echoes in our depths. In a wonderful manner conscience reveals that law which is fulfilled by love of God and neighbor....Christians are joined with the rest of people in the search for truth, and for the genuine solutions to the numerous problems which arise in the life of individuals and from social relationships. Hence the more right conscience holds sway, the more persons and groups turn aside from blind choice and strive to be guided by the objective norms of morality. Conscience frequently errs from invincible ignorance without losing its dignity. The same cannot be said for the person who cares but little for truth and goodness, nor for a conscience which by degrees grows practically sightless as a result of habitual sin.

It is important to note several dimensions of conscience as described above. First, conscience is referred to as "the sanctuary of the person" where one is alone with God and where God's voice echoes. It is the core of our being, our very deepest selves, a sacred place where we can meet the Holy One in prayer and attentive listening in order to discern the words of God and how we might best respond to the ever-present love of God. Second, in the depths of our conscience, we detect a law which holds us to obedience. Most generally, it summons or commands us to do good and avoid evil in whatever situation we find ourselves. It is essentially God's call in the depths of our being, in the depths of all human beings, to seek what is good and avoid doing what is evil, to respond out of love to God and neighbor. Third, what is right and good in a given situation may not always be apparent. The quote above points to the need for a *search* for truth and for genuine solutions to the moral issues that arise in daily life. This search is a primary role of conscience; it is the very work of conscience.

Finally, even though conscience is associated with the core of the individual, it is not an isolated reality. The search for moral truth is not something one does solely on one's own. Rather, it involves engagement with others. There is a social dimension to conscience. The individual, in the search to do what is right and good, should seek the moral wisdom of others, past and present. The moral wisdom of various communities is an essential ingredient of a healthy conscience. In addition, at times it is the community itself and not just the individual that is in search of what is right and good.

This book is meant to be one resource in the search to do what is right and to become good persons when facing specific moral challenges in the realm of health care. It offers moral wisdom drawn from the Catholic Christian tradition and from Church teaching. As such, it should prove helpful to individuals struggling to make informed moral choices about the health care issues discussed in its pages. But it could also be profitably employed in a group setting where individuals struggle together in the search for moral truth, who seek together to discern how God may be calling them to love with regard to a particular issue or in response to a specific situation. Such a "community of moral discourse" benefits from the lived experiences, professional competencies, varied perspectives, and moral wisdom of the group. Moral reflection is almost always best done in conversation with others, even if the ultimate decision is one's own to make.

The contributors to this volume take up six issues—stem cells, genetic testing, organ transplantation, end-of-life issues, advance health care directives, and medically administered nutrition and hydration.

Stem Cell Research

In the first chapter, M. Therese Lysaught discusses stem cell research. Before addressing the ethical concerns with human embryonic stem cell research, she provides an overview of what stem cells are and the different types and sources of stem cells. She then takes on the central issue in the embryonic stem cell debate—the moral status of the human embryo—and explores four positions, concluding with the one that reflects the Church's belief that human life is sacred and inviolable from the time of conception onward. This life, even in its earliest forms, ought not to be destroyed, even when there is a chance that it might benefit others. The moral status of the embryo is not the only moral issue associated with stem cell research, however. Lysaught explores other issues as well, including some that fall under the umbrella of "social justice." Here there is no specific Church teaching, but the Church's social justice tradition is operative, particularly its understanding of human dignity, equality, and distributive justice. In concluding her essay, Lysaught examines whether Catholics could licitly make use of therapies derived from embryonic stem cells in the event that they are ever developed.

Genetic Testing

In the second chapter, Carol Tauer examines genetic testing. More specifically, she considers various dimensions of genetic testing in adults, genetic testing for children and adolescents, and genetic testing associated with marital and reproductive decisions—such as premarital testing, carrier testing prior to pregnancy, and prenatal diagnosis once pregnancy has occurred. Among the moral concerns she considers are responses to positive test results, sharing of test results with family members, the appropriateness of testing children, and preventing the transmission of genetic diseases through marital and reproductive decisions. A cluster of fundamental values from the Catholic moral tradition frame her moral analysis of genetic testing, including respect for human dignity; our social nature and the responsibilities to others that it implies; our obligations to care for the vulnerable and marginalized; and responsible decision making, including responsible parenthood.

Organ Transplantation

Sister Patricia Talone discusses organ transplantation in the third chapter. She lays out Church teaching on organ donation generally and then examines the various types of organ donation—living donor and two types of dead donor—the critical role of informed consent (a concrete means of respecting human dignity) in organ donation, the buying and selling of organs, and brain death. Self-giving love is a dominant theme throughout the various parts of her discussion. This is buttressed by consideration of other key values—stewardship of our lives and bodies, the sanctity of human life, respect for human dignity, and solidarity with others.

End-of-Life Care

In the fourth chapter, Father Richard Sparks provides a brief overview of a number of aspects of end-of-life care—who should make treatment decisions and by what means, withholding and withdrawing treatment, palliative care, medically administered nutrition and hydration, the use of pain medication, and assisted suicide and euthanasia. This overview is prefaced with a critical discussion of what it means in the Catholic tradition to "respect life" in the face of life-threatening illness. As Father Sparks notes, the Catholic tradition does not require that human life be maintained at all costs, even though that life is deemed sacred and invaluable. Surely one is obliged to preserve human life, but one is only bound to do what is beneficial and what is reasonable. In the tradition and in Church teaching, this insight has been formulated in the principle of ordinary-extraordinary means or proportionate-disproportionate means. Respect for human life is a key theme in his discussion, but so are respect for human dignity and for the person in his or her totality, informed consent, the principle of ordinary-extraordinary means, and the principle of double effect (applied to the administration of pain medications).

Advance Health Care Directives

Father Mark Miller, in the next chapter, takes up and expands upon one of the issues addressed in the previous chapter—advance health care directives. Because this is such an important issue, it deserves a separate chapter. Father Miller explains the types of advance health care directives—instructional directives (living wills), the durable power of attorney for health care, and a combination of the two. A good deal of the chapter offers guidance in how to complete an advance health care directive. With regard to this issue, there is no specific Church teaching, though health care guidelines developed by the bishop's conferences of both the United States and Canada affirm advance health care directives so long as they do not conflict with Church teaching (for example, by requesting assisted suicide or euthanasia). Advance health care directives within the Catholic tradition are viewed as a legitimate exercise of the freedom of the individual to make decisions for himself or herself, often referred to as autonomy. Autonomy is one means of respecting human dignity and one's stewardship over one's life and body. In the Catholic tradition, however, this autonomy ought not be solely individualistic. It needs to take account of one's solidarity with others and, consequently, of one's responsibilities to them.

Medically Administered Nutrition and Hydration

In the final chapter, Michael Panicola also picks up on an issue briefly discussed in chapter five—medically administered nutrition and hydration. The heated controversy surrounding the Terri Schiavo case as well as the March 2004 speech of Pope John Paul II on the topic of medically administered nutrition and hydration and patients in a persistent vegetative state prompt an in-depth discussion. Panicola offers an overview of the centuries-old Catholic tradition on the duty to preserve life, examines some recent challenges to that tradition, and then comments on Pope John Paul II's March 2004 talk. He concludes with how Catholics might make decisions about feeding tubes in situations of life-threatening illness. As one might expect, the sanctity of life, the (limited) duty to preserve life, and the principle of ordinary and extraordinary means play a prominent role in his treatment of the issue.

Catholic Moral Tradition

In introducing each of the chapters of this book, I have highlighted values from the Catholic moral tradition that guide a moral analysis of the issue. Because these values are so important and because this volume is intended to provide guidance to Catholics making decisions about some of these issues, it is worth elaborating on some of the values. Hopefully, this will assist readers to better appeal to the values in their own moral reflection and decision making.

Sanctity of Human Life

This is a fundamental commitment of Catholicism—respect for human life from fertilization until natural death—because life, created in the image and likeness of God, is a gift of God. For these reasons, we have a duty to protect and preserve this sacred entity regardless of its stage or its quality. However, while it is indeed sacred, human life is not of absolute value. Consequently, not everything must be done to protect and preserve it. There are limits to that duty. We only need to do what is reasonable and what is beneficial. This gives rise to the principle of ordinary and extraordinary means which guides decisions about forgoing medical treatment at the end of life. Because of Catholicism's profound respect for human life, any direct and intended destruction of innocent human life is regarded as morally wrong—whether it is the destruction of early embryos to obtain stem cells, a fetus with a genetic mutation that will result in a severe genetic condition, or hastening the death of a terminal patient through physician-assisted suicide or euthanasia.

Human Dignity

Human dignity is one of the cornerstones of Catholic ethics. It maintains that every individual has an inherent and inalienable dignity or worth by the very fact that all are made in the image and likeness of God, redeemed by Christ, and destined for eternal communion with God. Intelligence, physical integrity and appearance, talents or lack thereof, race, social and economic status, and the like make no difference. Everyone has inherent value that cannot be given or taken away. Because of this we are called to respect this dignity in whatever situation we find ourselves interacting with others as individuals or communities. Human dignity, the sacredness of persons, is the basis of all moral obligation. It is because of this dignity that we ought to treat persons in certain ways and avoid treating them in other ways. Moral obligation calls us to respect human dignity and promote human well-being in ways that are appropriate to the specific situation. It is also human dignity that grounds basic human rights. The rights to food, clothing, shelter, education, employment, and health care are considered minimal requirements for living a decent human life, for achieving human flourishing.

Human dignity is central to all the issues dealt with in this volume. It is at issue in how we regard and treat those with genetic conditions, whether and how informed consent is observed in genetic testing and organ donation, how individuals exercise their autonomy in advance health care directives, and in the decisions we make for ourselves and for others at the end of life.

Relationality

While Catholicism has a profound regard for the individual and the dignity of the individual, it does not view the individual as isolated. Rather, it views human beings as social by nature—as existing in a variety of relationships and called to relationship. This fact of being in multiple relationships gives rise to responsibilities and obligations to others and to the common good. It is not just about the individual, but about the individual in his or her relationships. The individual must consider the social implications of his or her decisions, while society must consider the individual implications of policies and the like. Hence, Catholicism does not come down exclusively on the side of the individual or society, but attempts to maintain a very delicate balance between the two. This is sometimes expressed as the "individual-in-community." The social nature of human beings provides the moral basis for obligations and responsibilities to others, a responsibility to participate in society and to contribute to the common good.

Common good considerations come into play, for example, in how and where we allocate funds for stem cell research and genetic testing vis-à-vis other societal needs. It is present in a couple's reproductive decisions when, through testing, it becomes known that some of their future children are at high risk of having a severe genetic disability. And it is surely present in decisions about assisted suicide.

Justice

Taken together, human dignity and our social nature ground our obligations of justice. Justice is often described as giving others their due, that is, giving others what is owed them as human beings whether as individuals or as communities of individuals. With regard to individuals, we owe fairness in various exchanges and respect for basic human rights. With regard to society, we owe our contributions to that society and to the common good. The common good in Catholic social teaching is understood as the sum total of those economic, political, and social conditions necessary for human beings to enjoy their fundamental human rights and to flourish as human beings. In turn, society owes individuals. Society ought to structure itself so that individuals are able to participate in it and ought to distribute its goods and resources in ways that are equitable (which is not the same as equal). Some individuals may need to be given more in order to raise them up to a decent minimum level necessary for human flourishing.

Justice is particularly at issue in the matter of stem cell research. Is it just to devote billions of dollars to embryonic stem cell research that might one day result in therapies for various conditions and diseases when millions of individuals today are without basic health care? Are the benefits of genetic testing and of other genetic advances being made available in an equitable manner or are they being enjoyed by those who already benefit most from our health care system? How should human organs be allocated fairly?

Care for the Poor and Vulnerable

The Catholic moral tradition has always emphasized a special concern for those who are poor, vulnerable, and at the margins of society. This is because the God of the Hebrew scriptures revealed God's self as always on the side of the disadvantaged and marginalized. Likewise Jesus, the revelation of God, reached out to the sick, the marginalized, the poor, and sinners. Those on the margins should be of special concern to us. Their needs and their interests ought to have a certain primacy, especially in social policy decisions, and decisions that are made (or not made) should take account of the likely consequences upon the vulnerable. It is often said that the measure of a society is how it treats its poor and vulnerable.

What consideration, for example, is given to early (and vulnerable) human life in the embryonic stem cell debate? Is early human life being sacrificed now for the possible future benefit of others? How do the uninsured and underinsured fare when huge sums of public funds are directed toward embryonic stem cell research? Are those afflicted with genetic diseases discriminated against in various ways? How should we treat the vulnerable dying and those in persistent vegetative state?

The Totality of the Person

Besides its recognition of human dignity and our social nature, the Catholic moral tradition also regards the person in a holistic manner, that is, as a unity of body and spirit. Human beings are physical, psychological, spiritual, and social entities and ought not be reduced to any one dimension.

The notion of totality or a holistic approach to the person is critical in all dimensions of health care. In genetics, for example, there may be a tendency to reduce an individual to his or her physical integrity or genetic normalcy, forgetting the other core dimensions of the person. In many decisions about treatment, there is a tendency to focus on particular organ systems and what can be done to keep them going rather than looking at the effects of treatments on the person considered as a whole. This is especially important in end-of-life decision making about life-sustaining treatments. Often, they are capable of keeping life going, but with little or no benefit to the whole person.

Making Moral Decisions

The values that have been briefly outlined above are helpful guides to making moral decisions, but do not themselves provide answers. What else is needed? This depends on the complexity of the situation or issue. There are times when it is quite clear what is morally correct and what is not, and moral decisions come quite easily. In other instances, however, it is not so clear and coming to a decision requires a bit more work. The essays in this book provide information and moral guidance; they do not provide answers to specific situations. Only the individual(s) in those situations can make a decision of conscience as discussed previously. But while every moral decision ultimately rests with the conscience of the individual, one's conscience must be adequately formed. What does that entail?

Briefly, making a moral decision begins with acquiring adequate information about the issue at hand. Good ethics, it is said, begins with *good facts*. Unless we understand the issue in its various dimensions, it is less likely that we will make an appropriate moral response. With an adequate factual understanding as a basis, one moves on to examining key components of a moral decision. The first of these is the *intention*. What is it we are trying to achieve through a particular action? What is the goal or purpose of the action? When a physician administers morphine to a terminal cancer patient, for example, what is he or she trying to achieve? Why is he or she doing that? Presumably, it is to alleviate the patient's agonizing pain. This is a good intention. But it could also be to end the patient's life. This would be a bad intention which, in turn, would make the act morally wrong. For an act to be morally right, the intention must be good.

A second major consideration is the *act itself* or the *means*, that is, how I intend to achieve my goal. For an act to be morally right, not only must the intention be good, but the act (the means) must be congruent with the end or goal of one's action. There must be a "fit" between the two. The act or means must also be good. When looking at an action, one gets an initial impression about whether that action is good (donating one's organs after death) or harmful (destroying embryos to obtain stem cells) or neutral (undergoing prenatal diagnosis). In order for the means to fit a good end, one should choose a means that is either good or neutral.

Having said this, there are times when a good end or intention can justify a bad means. It may be that the bad means is the only way or the best way to achieve the end. The surgical removal of a uterus would generally not be considered as something good. However, it may be the only way to save the life of the woman whose uterus is cancerous. At other times, however, a good intention or end cannot justify a bad means because the means is so harmful to, or destructive, of persons. Even though the intention in embryonic stem cell research is good (to discover therapies that will alleviate much human suffering), the means (destruction of human embryos) is too evil to be justified. Destroying vulnerable early human life in order to relieve the suffering of others is a bad "fit." In this case, the means is incongruent with the end—in fact, it actually contradicts the end.

When considering the means or the action in question, it is essential also to take account of the likely *consequences* of the action—good and bad, short- and long-term. How will this action affect others? We should not choose an action that will have more harmful effects on others than good. The very purpose of our actions ought to be to achieve good, to respect human dignity, and to promote the well-being of others. Some actions will inevitably have harmful consequences, but these should not be dominant and they should be minimized as much as possible.

In addition to consequences, we also need to consider *alternatives*. Are there other and, perhaps, better ways to achieve one's goal or purpose? Are there actions that fit better with the intention? Do they produce fewer bad consequences or achieve greater good? The use of adult stem cells, for example, is an alternative to the use of embryonic stem cells and does not involve destroying human life or harming anyone. It is clearly a better fit with the goal of relieving human suffering.

Finally, one must consider *circumstances*, that is, the particularities of the situation that make it unique. The circumstances provide the texture of the situation. They are most often critical in determining the fit between the means and the end. Here we look at such things as *who*—who is performing the act and who is the recipient of it? *When* and *where* can also be as important as *what*—what is going on, what are the relevant facts of the situation?

Considering all these factors does not automatically lead to a conclusion. One must still make a judgment. One must still discern what course of action in the concrete situation best respects the dignity and promotes the well-being of the person or persons involved. We are not alone in making this judgment. There are many sources of moral wisdom available to us that provide guidance. Among them, for the Catholic Christian, are Scripture (though appealing to Scripture can be difficult), the Catholic theological and moral tradition, Church teaching, moral norms and principles (both religious and secular), the law, professional standards, human experience, and the wisdom of individuals and of the community, expressed verbally or in print. In the end, the most important source of moral guidance is God's Spirit. In prayerful reflection, open and attentive to God's presence, we take what we have gathered and discern how it is that God calls us to love in the situation at hand.

Acknowledgments

Hopefully, this book will be a source of moral guidance as well as helpful information to its readers. The book would not have seen the light of day were it not for Danny Michaels from Liguori Publications who originated this project and the six contributors, all friends and colleagues, who were willing to share their knowledge, insights, and moral wisdom. To them I am immensely grateful, as I am to the leadership of the Catholic Health Association of the United States—for its willingness to co-publish this book—and to my friends and colleagues, Scott McConnaha and Michael Panicola, the former for his editorial assistance and the latter for his helpful suggestions and advice along the way.

RON HAMEL, PHD
THE CATHOLIC HEALTH ASSOCIATION
OF THE UNITED STATES
JANUARY 2006

CHAPTER 1

Making Decisions about Embryonic Stem Cell Research

M. Therese Lysaught, PhD

The controversy over human embryonic stem cell research (HESCR) has raged, now, for seven years with no sign of abating. Legislative initiatives crowd state ballots. Human cloning moves forward with proposals for international research consortia. Promises, accusations, hope, and hype are bandied about in the press. Positions seem intractably staked out, with little hope of resolution.

How are faithful Catholics to navigate this rapidly changing scientific and legislative landscape? This chapter is designed to help with that challenge. I begin by providing a brief background on stem cells. I then review the debate on one of the central issues–the moral status of the human embryo and then discuss other ethical considerations that must be taken into account in assessing claims about HESCR in the media and in decisions about federal and state legislative initiatives. While these are currently the main issues, another critical question could emerge if therapies are eventually developed from HESCR. Patients may one day be faced with a decision about whether to use such therapies. This, too, I will consider.

Stem Cells—Embryonic and Otherwise

Human Embryonic Stem Cells

What *is* a stem cell? Stem cells form in the earliest stages of human development after a fertilized egg begins to divide. After seven or eight divisions, the egg is known as a blastocyst—a sphere made up of two types of cells. One type forms a well-defined outer layer destined to become the placenta and the remaining cells cluster together off to one side of the blastocyst. These cells are all the same. That is, they have not started to "differentiate" or become the different tissues that make up the human body and that will eventually develop into a fetus. These "undifferentiated" cells are human embryonic stem cells.

The controversy around human embryonic stem cells began in November 1998 (though researchers have been working with embryonic stem cells from different mammals since 1981) when two researchers—John Gearhart at Johns Hopkins University and James Thompson at the University of Wisconsin—announced that they had figured out how to obtain human embryonic stem cells and make them live and grow in their labs for up to nine months. Thompson derived his cells from week-old human embryos produced by in vitro fertilization. Gearhart isolated his from fetuses aborted at five to nine weeks (Actually, the cells isolated by Gearhart are technically called embryonic germ cells. They are precursors of sperm and egg cells and are very similar to stem cells.) Both Thompson and Gearhart demonstrated that human embryonic stem cells (and germ cells) could be directed to "differentiate" into the three basic types of embryonic tissue and, from there, into any of the over two hundred types of cells in the human body.

Because they can develop into any type of tissue in the human body, human embryonic stem cells, it is argued, have potential to provide significant scientific and medical benefits. Scientifically, these cells would be ideal for studying human embryonic development, particularly developmental disorders. Medical researchers also anticipate a number of clinical applications. They imagine the possibility of growing organs to use for transplantation as well as tissue to replace damaged tissue, potentially providing therapies for diseases like Parkinson's, juvenile diabetes, Alzheimer's, congestive heart failure, spinal cord injury, arthritis, muscular dystrophy, kidney disease, liver disease, and more. These cells could also be used for testing pharmaceuticals and other chemicals to see if they are toxic or effective.

Cloning

In the process described above, stem cells are obtained from embryos created by "in vitro fertilization" (also known as IVF). These embryos are either specifically created for research or, more frequently, are obtained from fertility clinics. In the latter situation, the embryos are created by couples facing reproductive obstacles who desire to have children. Most often the IVF process results in more embryos than can be implanted, so some are "left over." Many researchers see these "surplus" IVF embryos as a rich source of stem cells.

When used for pharmaceutical testing or studying human development, the source of the stem cells is not terribly important. For purposes of potential therapeutic application, however, the source can be critical. With stem cells as with any other type of tissue or organ transplantation, rejection can occur. Consequently, much of the interest has shifted to cloning as a source of stem cells. Cloning, it is argued, would provide human embryonic stem cells tailored to individual patients, thereby eliminating the risk of tissue rejection.

Cloning is now often referred to as "somatic cell nuclear transfer," abbreviated SCNT. To make a clone, researchers must obtain an ovum and remove the nucleus (the center of the cell where most of the genes reside). Then a cell (for example, a skin cell) is taken from the body of a different adult, in this case the patient. Since it comes from the patient's body, it is referred to as a "somatic" cell (*somatic* meaning "body"). The nucleus of this skin cell is also removed and then injected or "transferred" into the enucleated ovum. The ovum is then stimulated with an electrical charge, chemicals, and hormones, and the materials from the two different cells fuse. The ovum now has a full complement of genes and it begins to act like it has been fertilized. It begins to divide and grow and become an embryo.

At this point in the cloning process, two things could happen. The embryo could be implanted into the uterus of a woman and brought to term. The President's Council on Bioethics names this process "cloning to produce children." Alternatively, the embryo could be used as a source of stem cells that would be an exact genetic match to the tissue of the patient who donated the skin cell. Therefore, if these stem cells could be used to grow tissues or organs or derive other therapies, the products generated from the stem cells would not be rejected by the patient. The President's Council names this process "cloning for biomedical research." The President's Council prefers these two phrases over those more commonly heard in the media—particularly, "reproductive cloning and therapeutic cloning"—which they believe mask any attempt to "solve moral questions by artful redefinition."

Adult Stem Cells
Embryos are not the only source of stem cells. Although somewhat more difficult to locate and isolate, stem cells are found in all tissues in the human body—in the liver, bone marrow, brain, and so on. Stem cells, as noted earlier, give rise to all these different tissues. But when they do, reservoirs of undifferentiated stem cells remain in

order to replenish tissue over our lifetime and to repair damage to tissue when it occurs. These stem cells can be culled out of the various tissues in which they reside and then cultivated and used for therapeutic purposes. Although they are found in infants as well, these cells are referred to as "adult stem cells."

Adult stem cells have been used therapeutically for over forty years. What used to be referred to as a "bone marrow transplant" is now referred to as a "stem cell transplant," because the therapeutic agent in the transplant consists in stem cells in the bone marrow. The therapeutic potential of adult stem cells has also been demonstrated in the treatment of other diseases, including diabetes, advanced kidney cancer, heart disease, and more. Many clinical trials are currently underway to assess the therapeutic effectiveness of adult stem cells against a variety of conditions. That adult stem cell research has advanced to and through the stage of clinical trials is highly significant.

The flexibility of adult stem cells is as yet unclear. Until recently, it was believed that adult stem cells were limited in their ability to be transformed into any type of tissue in the body. It was believed that they were too specialized—for example, blood-forming stem cells could only form blood cells; liver stem cells could only form liver cells, and so on. As more research has been conducted on adult stem cells, however, it appears that they may be far more flexible than previously thought. Adult stem cells offer patients the same advantage as that proposed for cloning—they are an exact genetic match to the patient, eliminating the risk of rejection.

Stem Cells from Umbilical Cord Blood

One final source of stem cells is umbilical cord blood. The blood in the umbilical cord and placenta is unique because it contains large numbers of blood-forming stem cells. For almost twenty years, cord blood has been used in lieu of bone marrow in what is now recognized to be stem cell transplants, as noted above. Cord blood banks have grown over time, recruiting expectant mothers to donate their baby's umbilical cord blood for research and transplantation. Since the advent of interest in human embryonic stem cells, the stem cells from cord blood are being studied in a new way as an alternative source of stem cells for developing treatments for life-threatening diseases.

With almost four million babies born every year in the U.S. alone, cord blood represents an extraordinary resource for obtaining stem cells. Again, as in the case of cloning, these stem cells would be an exact genetic match to the donor (the baby), but could also be used to treat nonrelated patients. Cord blood banks are currently growing, nationally and internationally.

The Moral Status of the Embryo

The debate on the morality of HESCR centers, of course, on the destruction of human embryos. For many who consider embryos to be living human beings, this in and of itself raises insurmountable moral barriers to this type of research. Others, however, view embryos differently. Four primary positions have emerged on this question.

Embryos Are Not Human Life

A first position denies that the blastocyst qualifies as "human" life. Some view the blastocyst as simply human tissue, a cluster of cells, insufficiently organized to qualify as a "living being." Others argue that the mode of origination makes a difference. Since, in the case of in vitro fertilization and especially SCNT (somatic cell nuclear transfer—cloning), the natural process of human fertilization is bypassed, the blastocyst or embryo should not be considered the same as other embryos. SCNT, rather than creating a new human life, simply "extends and expands the donor's cell mass" and should therefore be seen as an extension of the donor to be used as she or he wishes. Often, the products of these technological processes are referred to as "clonates" or "recombinant embryos." Thus, if the embryo is simply human tissue or is relocated into a different category of identity, the moral question simply goes away. As the President's Council noted, however, one should always exercise caution in the face of new language.

Embryos Are Not Human Persons

A second position grants that the blastocyst qualifies as human life but argues that because it lacks certain characteristics (most often, consciousness and self-awareness), it does not count as a human *person*. Embryos may certainly have the *potential* to become human persons, it is argued, but since that potential is not yet realized, they cannot yet be accorded the same respect due a person and do not have the rights of a person.

Similarly, some Catholic moral theologians argue that the blastocyst is too undeveloped to be counted as a human person. Before it implants (ten to fourteen days after fertilization), a blastocyst is still open to the possibility of splitting in two—in other words, of becoming twins. As long as a blastocyst is open to this possibility, an important precondition of personal identity—namely, individuality—is not yet established. Thus, they argue that the blastocyst cannot be considered a human person and therefore, although it deserves "respect," it does not deserve the level of respect that must be accorded to embryos that have been implanted (rarely is there any specification of what such "respect" concretely entails). Therefore, embryos can potentially be used or treated in ways that other human beings who have attained the status of "persons" cannot.

Human Life Versus Human Life

A third position theoretically accepts that human embryos might rightly be considered living human beings but then takes a utilitarian line of reasoning. Typically it weighs the loss of a minimal number of human embryos against the "millions" (the number often given) of human lives that could potentially be saved or helped should HESCR and cloning bear therapeutic fruit. This position emerges especially in relation to the fate of "surplus" IVF embryos. Many argue that since these embryos are going to be discarded anyway, they should be used for research and the development of therapies that could (theoretically) relieve the suffering of other human beings. The moral benefits of the research, they argue, outweigh the moral costs.

Many proposals put forward in favor of HESCR almost universally draw the line at fourteen days. But importantly, once those arguments are deemed acceptable—namely, that embryos are not "persons" because they lack some characteristic—then that line becomes quite fragile. What is to prevent that line from being extended into the fetal or even preterm stages if it were found that cells at those stages are more usable for therapies? How will one hold the line against this type of argumentation if one has admitted its acceptability elsewhere, especially against the overriding imperative of relieving suffering?

Embryos Are Living Human Subjects

A fourth position, one that shapes official Catholic teaching, argues that blastocysts and embryos are indeed living human subjects with a right to life whose dignity is to be respected from fertilization to death. This position holds that at conception a unique individual is created, one with a unique genetic endowment that organizes and guides the expression of both its shared human identity and its own individual character. That which gives it its own unique identity is already "realized" in its genetic makeup. This position is radically egalitarian, seeing each human life equal in worth and dignity to other human life, regardless of one's social, intellectual, or physical condition. Moreover, it highlights the fundamental Christian conviction captured in the important principle of the "preferential option for the poor"—that we are to provide *greater* protections toward those who are weak, vulnerable, and not self-sufficient, not less. Thus, research that destroys human embryos is gravely immoral, regardless of the positive outcomes or the intention to help others.

Further Moral Considerations

The concern for the dignity of the human person does not exhaust the moral analysis. Rather, it interfaces with other moral considerations that further express the Church's commitment to human life and dignity. I shall now consider some of these.

The Church's Commitment to Healing and Research

The Catholic Church has long been at the forefront of the human obligation to heal and care for the sick. From the gospels onward, healing has been recognized as something central to the activity of Christ, to the presence of God in the world, and therefore to the work of the Church and to the meaning of Christian discipleship. This commitment is embodied in the extensive network of Catholic hospitals and health care-related facilities worldwide.

Moreover, the Church has long supported and promoted scientific research for the benefit of humanity through various Vatican offices that focus on questions of science and technology as well as through the extensive network of Catholic colleges, universities, and medical schools around the globe. While the Church has traditionally encouraged investigation in the fields of medicine and biology, with the goal of curing diseases and improving the quality of life for all, it does maintain that such research and clinical care must be respectful of the dignity of the human being.

Thus, faith and rigorous science and medicine are not mutually exclusive. Nonetheless, pursuit of healing and research must be situated within a broader moral framework that can direct these tools toward the common good. Without this, they become ends-in-themselves, a form of idolatry. The Church's position on HESCR, therefore, must be situated within the broader context of its longstanding and ongoing commitment to quality medical care and rigorous research.

Risks of Harm

In evaluating any new, experimental interventions one must also consider the balance between the probable benefit versus probable harm. But this must be done with care. As we have seen, a utilitarian view suggests that the harm done to embryos is outweighed by the potential benefit to those stricken with diseases. Here the burdens or harms fall on one population (the embryos that are "sacrificed") and the benefits accrue to another population (future patients). History has recognized the dangers of calculating harm and benefit in this way. Generally, harms are permitted to fall on populations that lack power or voice, while the benefits accrue to those most similar to the ones making the calculation.

Furthermore, given the probability that therapeutic applications, if they occur at all, are likely to take three to five decades to develop, the harm/benefit analysis is unbalanced. The "harms" (if one counts the destruction of human embryos as a serious moral consideration) are real harms being incurred now, while the possible benefits remain future and hypothetical. They may well never be realized. Those who are sensitive to the issue of who bears the harms—a serious justice issue and one which does not occur with adult stem cells—would counsel against HESCR.

Profits and Products

Over the past thirty years or so, biotech research has come to be fueled much more by profits and commercialization than by altruistic motives. Consequently, no HESCR initiative can be assessed apart from considerations of the commodification and commercialization of human tissue—that is, of turning human body parts into products to be traded, objects to be bought and sold.

Interestingly, much of the controversy over HESCR since 1998 has concerned funding, particularly the use of federal funds, that is, tax-payer dollars. As with all new biotech developments, one must ask who stands to profit? Profitability is clearly a primary driving force behind this research. The company that funded Thomson's and Gearhart's work (Geron), for example, now holds an exclusive license on their techniques. Those who wish to develop stem cells for research or potential therapies have to pay Geron a fee. Typically, with each new step of research along the way, there is a rush to patent, even when the research is publicly funded. Ironically, those who "donate" the "raw materials" (eggs and sperm) to make cloned embryos or those who donate their "surplus" IVF embryos cannot be paid (though egg donors can be compensated for their "inconvenience"). Apart from the profit motive and the related commercialization of human tissues is the issue of commodification. Most of the legislative efforts that have been advanced in favor of cloning propose that the manufacture of embryos as material for research or therapy be overseen by the FDA, thereby classifying human embryos as marketable "biological products." What does such language assume and convey? How is our understanding of nascent human life—as well as the rest of human life—transformed when we change our terms and begin speaking of embryos as "products"?

If we assume that HESCR or cloning for research actually becomes clinically useful, providing benefits to "millions" of patients as is often promised, the process of creation (whether cloned or created through IVF), destruction, and trading of nascent human life would need to be institutionalized in a systematic and large-scale manner. Human lives would by necessity become products of a manufacturing technique. How would this affect the dignity of the human person broadly speaking? Would it be possible to treat one embodiment of human life in this manner without it affecting how we view human life as a whole? That HESCR is so deeply implicated in the profit motive and commodification raises serious questions for its impact on the dignity of human life in general and, therefore, on the common good.

Social Justice

The Catholic social justice tradition raises another set of questions, as Joseph Cardinal Bernardin reminds us, "life" issues and social justice issues are parts of a single piece. While not unique to stem cell research, one must always consider the deep contradiction in our culture, that is, when so many resources are mustered to gain funding for one particular initiative—one that may take decades to bear fruit—while we lack the political will to make basic, real therapies available to people who need them now.

In November 2004, the people of California passed a proposition to fund embryonic stem cell research with a three billion dollar bond issue that will actually cost them six billion dollars in principal and interest. Yet seven million Californians and forty-five million Americans have no health insurance coverage. Twelve million children in the U.S. live in poverty. Worldwide, twenty-eight thousand children per day—over ten million children per year—die from preventable diseases. One person dies every six seconds from a disease for which we have vaccines. Is it just to redirect resources of this magnitude away from real needs that could be met now with readily available resources to fund a line of research that might never bear fruit? Against the claim of proponents of HESCR that it will one day relieve enormous human suffering stands a sea of real, immediate human suffering that could easily be addressed with readily available interventions. Moreover, should HESCR ever bear therapeutic fruit, will these same children who are dying in the millions, these same people who lack access to vaccines or drugs, have access to high-tech therapies developed from HESCR or cloned embryos? Probably not. We must ask: Is HESCR or human cloning the best place to invest if economic resources are limited? What will go unfunded so that HESCR can move forward?

A second social justice question concerns the source of the raw materials for this research. IVF and human cloning require human eggs. Current legislation requires that embryos and ova be "donated" for research. Women cannot be paid for them, though they can be compensated (approximately $2,400) for the "inconvenience" egg donation entails, which is considerable. With the goal being to maximize efficiency and harvest as many eggs as possible from each round, is there a risk that women might be prescribed excessive doses of fertility drugs so that they can produce more eggs?

In addition, were HESCR or cloning to bear therapeutic fruit, there will be a large-scale need for ova. It is not farfetched to imagine that underprivileged women in the U.S. or abroad might find the "compensation" offered for egg donation hard to resist. And should egg harvesting go "off shore," as has so much industrial production in recent years, it is likely that any safeguards that are in place in the U.S. will be pushed aside and any compensation offered will mirror the dollar a day that foreign workers make in free-trade zones. It is extremely difficult to enforce ethical guidelines in the face of the overwhelming pressure to create results, to fulfill the scientific imperative. These social justice questions should raise some of the most critical (though unfortunately often overlooked) concerns for the practice of HESCR.

The Use of Therapies Derived from Human Embryonic Stem Cells

One final question must be asked. In the event that human embryonic stem cell research or cloning bear therapeutic fruit, would it be morally licit for a Catholic to use those therapies? If, in other words, one has a therapy derived using means considered to be immoral by the Church, is the use of that therapy then likewise considered morally problematic?

Appropriation and Complicity

The answer to this question will depend in large part on the mode and infrastructure of production of such therapies. While patients in these cases might not be directly or even indirectly involved with the wrongdoing itself, what moral judgment can be offered about those who knowingly "appropriate" the outcomes of evil actions? If someone were to give you a pile of money that you knew had been robbed from a bank, would you not be "ratifying" the wrong done if you kept and used it? Would the use of therapies, especially the regular use of therapies in a chronic condition, render one complicit in some way? When I benefit over and over again from a wrong while simply ignoring the wrong itself, do I entrench myself in an established relationship with that wrong whether I approve of it or not?

Within the Catholic tradition, levels of complicity are determined in part by the degree of distance one can achieve between one's own action and the wrongdoing. Such distance can be achieved in a number of ways. One is time. If two actions are separated by a significant amount of time, the later one may be justifiable or, at least, the moral taint may be minimized. A second is the degree of separation or the number of steps intervening between a present act and a prior act. A third is whether or not the original evil act or practice is ongoing. A fourth is whether refusal to participate in a set of practices due to their link with prior evil would, if practiced broadly, effectively unravel the social fabric and be detrimental to the common good.

Given the current status of stem cell research, it is doubtful whether one could establish sufficient distance between any therapies and the destruction of embryos. Researchers continue to develop new stem cell lines. Furthermore, if therapies are ever developed, their utilization would fuel the ongoing practice of stem cell derivation; it would create a demand, and given the probable high cost of these interventions, it would likewise create a market. Indeed, it would require and create an industrial-level institutionalization of the destruction of embryos, thereby encouraging, providing a supportive alliance, or even lending legitimacy to the destruction of human life based on the premise of healing. The only reason for destroying the embryos is to gain the stem cells and there would be few intervening steps between the embryo and the therapeutically applied tissues.

Some argue that to shun this research will undercut the common good by preventing the development of therapies that could benefit large numbers of people. At this juncture, the benefits are theoretical and will most likely not be produced for decades, if at all. Many an embryo will be sacrificed from which no good will come. If the goods are not immediate, there remains the question of alternatives. Given the promise of adult stem cells and cord blood, the active pursuit of these alternatives would not only avoid the issue of complicity entirely but would provide a powerful counter-practice that would largely render moot the topic at hand.

Conclusion

One positive outcome of the debate over HESCR that emerged in 2005 is that some scientists have been earnestly looking for alternative ways to develop embryonic stem cells without destroying human life. Some are doing this simply because they do not want their work to be caught up in controversy. Others are doing it because they care deeply about respecting human life. Within the past year, two possibilities have been put forward. One proposes to limit current pre-implantation genetic techniques in order to make possible the remove of a single stem cell from an embryo without destroying it. Another suggests a mechanism similar to SCNT, but altering the ovum ahead of time so that when fused with the adult body cell, it has no possibility of ever developing into an embryo. These alternatives may raise their own issues, but it is heartening to see that science can indeed respond to moral argument and can then do what it does best—creatively pursue new and less morally grave avenues to achieve worthy goals.

In the end, addressing HESCR requires the virtue of prudence. Most forms of moral reasoning, including Catholic moral reasoning, hold that if one is presented with two courses of action, one of which is morally less controversial or noncontroversial, one ought to choose that option. It may well be more complicated, less efficient, more time-consuming, and so on, but generally, prudence would counsel the morally safer course. Thus, alternative sources of stem cells provide a noncontroversial way to pursue the real goods promised by regenerative medicine. They also provide more realistic hope for therapeutic benefit.

The Christian tradition has long held that the cultivation of one virtue simultaneously engages the cultivation of others. In the case of HESCR, we must remain attentive to the role of virtues in our discernment and relationship to this practice. The virtue of honesty will call us to "fair and accurate" language in our descriptions of these processes and entities. The virtue of hope will push us to foster realistic hope rather than raising false hope through hype. The virtue of justice will sharpen our radars for how these technologies impact the poor and vulnerable. The virtue of fortitude may well be required should one decide to choose against a therapy that could save one's own life yet would enmesh one too deeply in a morally problematic infrastructure. And so on.

The Christian tradition has much to offer those seeking to navigate the often confusing terrain of HESCR. Through a richer understanding of the moral life, of the human person, of moral analysis, and its deep commitment to healing and knowledge, the Christian tradition provides a sound and hopeful way forward.

Questions for Discussion

1. Do you agree with the Church's and the author's position that the destruction of human embryos to obtain stem cells is morally wrong, even when done in the hope of eventually relieving human suffering? Why? Why not?

2. What view of the moral status of the embryo do you hold? Why?

3. Do you believe it is morally permissible to destroy "spare embryos," that is, frozen embryos left over from in vitro fertilization, in order to obtain stem cells?

4. Do you think that too much money is being spent on embryonic stem cell research when that money could be used to provide basic health care to many people who are without it?

5. Do you agree with the author that if therapies are ever developed from human embryonic stem cell research, it would not be ethical to use them?

For Further Reading

Branick, V., and M. Therese Lysaught, "Stem Cell Research: Licit or Complicit?" *Health Progress* 80, no. 5 (September–October 1999): 37–42.

Do No Harm: The Coalition of Americans for Research Ethics. For an organization of scientists opposed to human embryonic stem cell research, see http://www.stemcellresearch.org.

Pontifical Academy for Life, "Declaration on the Production and the Scientific and Therapeutic Use of Human Embryonic Stem Cells" (August 2000). See http://www.vatican.va.

President's Council on Bioethics at http://www.bioethics.gov.

Shannon, Thomas A., and James J. Walter. *The New Genetic Medicine: Theological and Ethical Reflections.* Lanham, Md.: Rowman & Littlefield, 2003, 120–160.

Snow, Nancy, ed. *Stem Cell Research: New Frontiers in Science and Ethics.* Notre Dame, Ind.: University of Notre Dame Press, 2003.

United States Conference of Catholic Bishops. For more information on adult stem cell research and other questions about stem cells, see the Web site of the USCCB at http://www.nccbuscc.org/prolife.

CHAPTER 2

Making Decisions about Genetic Testing

Carol A. Tauer, PhD

S uppose your father recently died of Huntington's, an adult-onset disease. You are thinking of having your four children tested for the Huntington's gene so that you can invest your limited funds in the education of the children who are free of the threat of this disease. However, you wonder if such a plan is fair to the children.

Or suppose that your extended family has a history of breast and ovarian cancer. After genetic testing confirms your risk, you are considering preventive removal of your breasts and ovaries, but you are uncertain as to whether this surgery is morally permissible.

Or imagine that a family member wants you to participate in testing to identify a particular disease mutation that may be present in your family. While you would like to cooperate, you suspect that she is interested in identifying the mutation so that if she becomes pregnant, she can have her fetus tested.

These three scenarios illustrate the sorts of decisions that many of us will have to face in relation to genetic testing. The field of genomics has made important advances that promise great benefits, but genetic progress also gives rise to moral, ethical, interpersonal, and social challenges. Some of these challenges, particularly regarding prenatal genetic diagnosis, are related to longstanding concerns about the protection of fetal life. Other challenges, such as issues arising in the genetic testing of adults, are newer.

Catholics may reasonably ask what the Church has said on these matters. While it is well known that the Church prohibits abortion based on identification of a fetal defect, the Church's positions on other genetic issues are not as familiar. In fact, on the majority of ethical issues arising from genetic testing, the Church has been fairly silent, recognizing that in most cases the persons involved must weigh the pros and cons and come to their own decisions.

We are not left without guiding principles, however. Three principles are relevant to genetic decisions:

- The *principle of human dignity* requires that we respect every human life, its value and potential, and that we avoid practices that discriminate among humans on the basis of perceived or actual limitations.
- The *principle of relationality* requires a balance between the needs and wishes of an individual, on the one hand, and on the other, the responsibilities of that individual within the family and the larger community.
- The *principle of solidarity* reminds us of our obligation to care for those who are most needy, physically, psychologically, or economically, thus ensuring that all are able to benefit from medical and genomic advances.

In applying these three principles, the individual is governed by the *principle of responsibility*. Faced with a difficult decision, what course of action would a well-informed, thoughtful, responsible person pursue? For most decisions regarding genetic testing, there is no one answer that applies to every individual or every family. While an individual must seek information and is often advised to have professional counseling, in the end no one can tell him or her what to do. The person directly involved is morally responsible for choosing among the available options.

This chapter will first explore genetic testing related to health concerns of adults and the use of testing for children and adolescents. Second, it will discuss genetic testing in relation to reproductive decisions, identifying ways in which such testing can be acceptable under Church teaching. Last, the chapter will review the growing field of pharmacogenomics, the use of genetics in the development and prescribing of drugs.

Genetic Testing for Adults

Genetic tests identify individuals who are likely, or more likely than the average person, to develop a particular disease—information similar to that found in one's family history. However, genetic test results are often regarded (perhaps mistakenly) as somewhat more sensitive and private than family history.

Genetic testing in adults can be directed to a variety of purposes. For example, if one is already experiencing symptoms of a particular disease, then a *diagnostic* genetic test may be used to verify the cause of the symptoms. A *presymptomatic* test may indicate the presence of a gene for a particular genetic disease such as Huntington's, though symptoms may not yet be evident. A *predictive* or *predispositional* test may identify a higher-than-average probability of developing a common disease, for example, breast or colon cancer.

All of these uses of genetic tests can be integrated into good medical care and can be provided in ways that are completely consistent with Catholic teaching. As the American bishops note in their document, "Critical Decisions: Genetic Testing and Its Implications," the Church "welcomes testing when it functions as an extension of sound medical practice." Diagnostic genetic tests are simply another instrument for identifying possible causes for a patient's symptoms. Predictive tests can be used to plan treatment regimens that may prevent the predicted disease from occurring, or they may help the individual patient make life-altering decisions regarding career, marriage, and parenthood.

Criteria for Decisions about Testing

While diagnostic tests raise no unique issues, both presymptomatic and predictive tests require the individual to weigh carefully the benefits and risks of testing. Three considerations are particularly important: (1) family history; (2) possible responses to positive test results; and (3) implications for relationships and the family system.

Family History

The family health history of an individual provides significant information about that person's risk factors for many diseases, including breast and colon cancer, heart disease, stroke, and type-2 diabetes. Family history is essential as a criterion for decisions about genetic testing. Apart from some newborn screening, there is essentially no disease for which genetic screening of the entire population is recommended. Only when a person has a family history suggesting elevated risk would a genetic test be proposed. Despite some direct-to-consumer advertising that may encourage members of the general population to seek genetic testing, such testing is discouraged by medical providers. Without a family history of susceptibility to a disease, genetic testing may be seriously misleading and, in fact, may produce a number of false positive results leading to unnecessary follow-up testing and useless treatment.

Responses to Positive Test Results

The second consideration in making a decision to undergo genetic testing is whether something effective can be done if the test is positive.

For some diseases that a test might predict, there are possible preventive strategies. If genetic tests indicate an elevated risk of breast cancer, for example, frequent mammograms may be recommended. Or tests indicating an increased risk of colon cancer may lead to a recommendation for regular colonoscopies and modifications in diet.

Perhaps the most controversial response to a positive predictive test is prophylactic or preventive removal of body parts or organs. For example, this procedure is most common when the risk is breast cancer, where studies have shown that bilateral mastectomy and also oophorectomy (ovary removal) are highly effective in preventing breast or ovarian cancer. Removal of the colon in early adult life is another procedure that is sometimes recommended for a particular type of hereditary susceptibility to colon cancer that involves excessive production of colon polyps.

In the latter situation, the colon could be considered to be abnormal or unhealthy, so surgery would involve removal of a diseased organ and would not be morally controversial. But what about the other case—removal of breasts and/or ovaries that may be at risk but are not yet diseased?

Specific statements on this topic have been made by the Church's teaching authority. In a 1953 address to a medical conference, Pope Pius XII spoke on "The Removal of a Healthy Organ." He proposed three conditions, which appear to be satisfied for preventive mastectomy or oophorectomy for a woman whose family history and/or genetic testing indicate a highly elevated cancer risk.

[First,] the continued presence…of a particular organ within the whole organism…constitutes a menace to it; next, this damage…can be measurably lessened by the mutilation [sic] in question…; finally, one must be reasonably certain that the negative effect…will be compensated for by the positive effect: elimination of danger to the whole organism.

Given the fact that removal of the ovaries also has the effect of ending the fertility of the woman, one might ask whether any additional conditions apply to this type of preventive surgery. Pius XII addresses this point in the context of a woman whose health or life would be threatened by a pregnancy because of unhealthy organs (kidneys, heart, lungs, and so forth) other than the ovaries. In this case, he asserts that removal of the ovaries would not be justified since they are not the organs that present a threat to the woman.

In the situation we are discussing, however, it is specifically the ovaries (as well as the breasts) that endanger the organism as a whole. Thus their removal appears to be justified by the conditions enunciated by Pope Pius XII. In actuality, the question of ending fertility may not arise, since the woman considering preventive oophorectomy will often be past her reproductive years.

Lack of Preventive Strategies

While the likelihood of developing a predicted genetically linked disease can often be lessened by preventive measures, in many cases no preventive strategies are available. For example, there is no proven prevention for Alzheimer's disease, although staying active both mentally and physically may offer a modest benefit. There is no means of preventing Huntington's in a person who carries the gene for this disease. While the age of onset of symptoms and their severity differ from person to person, at present there is no way to affect these factors.

If there is essentially nothing that can be done in response to a positive genetic test, is there any reason to choose to have such a test? Some people who have a family history of a particular disease may consider it more beneficial simply to know, rather than not to know, what their prognosis is. A person considering a test for this reason needs to explore benefits, risks, and possible consequences of testing after full consideration of pros and cons. In the case of Huntington's, for example, clinics report that persons who come for testing often do not return to receive test results, indicating a high degree of ambivalence.

However, when a person is faced with life-altering decisions related to genetic risk, then the person may have a responsibility to be tested. Perhaps the most crucial decisions in this regard are whether to marry and whether to have children. A person with the Huntington's gene would have a 50 percent chance of passing that gene to each child. Often the risk is less; for example, if someone is a carrier for a gene mutation related to cystic fibrosis (CF), then the possibility of having a child with CF depends on whether one's partner is a carrier for a similar mutation. Yet there may still be a responsibility to have accurate information on one's genetic status as a basis for informed decisions.

Implications of Testing for Family Members

Genetic testing of an individual has implications not only for that person, but for family members and relatives. One's siblings, children, and even parents may be affected by testing and test results.

What is the extent of an individual's responsibility to inform relatives of genetic risk and genetic test results? There are several criteria to consider: (1) how closely the person is related, thus how likely to share genetic risk; (2) whether it is probable that the person would want the information; (3) whether treatment or prevention is available; and (4) whether life decisions may be affected.

Relatives might well want to know about a risk of hereditary hemochromatosis, for example, since further tests may indicate the advisability of treatment that is known to be effective. On the other hand, little is gained by informing relatives that one has a gene that suggests a high risk for developing Alzheimer's. The prediction is highly uncertain and there is no proven preventive strategy.

Between these two rather clear cases would fall predictive tests for breast cancer. Most members of high-risk families probably know they are at risk, since some individuals will already have had breast or ovarian cancer or both. Notification of a positive genetic test is likely not to be a surprise to family members, and it may be useful information for others who are thinking of being tested. In many situations the presence of a particular deleterious mutation within a family may be important in evaluating the significance of genetic tests of other family members. Thus it may be helpful if a woman who does not wish to know her own genetic status is willing to provide test results to assist others as a family pattern is studied.

The principle of relationality suggests that in making decisions about genetic testing, the individual ought to consider the ramifications of a positive test for other family members. Physicians and genetic counselors generally advise a client to notify affected relatives, but if the person chooses not to do so, professionals will almost never override that choice. However, there is some uncertainty as to whether a physician or other professional could be held legally liable if a relative were seriously harmed for lack of information that was withheld from him or her.

A person has a particular obligation to inform a potential marriage partner of known genetic risks. Without such disclosure, the marriage partner is entering into a covenant under false pretenses. Deliberate deception might even contribute to grounds for an annulment if the spouse later became aware of the deception.

In view of one's responsibility for the welfare of one's own children, it is also essential to inform them of hereditary conditions and risks in the family. Of course, the appropriate time for such disclosure varies from child to child and is ordinarily inadvisable until the child has reached maturity or until treatment or preventive strategies are indicated.

Cooperation with Unacceptable Applications

What about situations where an individual believes that genetic information may be used by a relative in a morally unacceptable way? In particular, what if one suspects that information may be used in order to request prenatal testing of a fetus, possibly leading to an abortion?

In answering this question, it would be appropriate to follow the lead of genetic testing services in Catholic institutions as well as the approach of pro-life genetic research scientists. Catholic institutions offer genetic services, including prenatal testing, knowing that couples and potential parents have many acceptable alternatives for use of this information, though they might also make a morally unacceptable choice. A scientist who discovers the gene for a disease knows it might eventually be used for prenatal testing leading to abortion, but this possibility is not an adequate argument for opposing all genetic research. For example, scientist Jerome Lejeune, an abortion opponent, discovered the chromosomal anomaly for Down syndrome and for many other birth defects. While publishing these results, he consistently opposed the use of his discoveries for selective abortion.

Unless a relative asks for information explicitly in order to determine whether to abort a pregnancy, the individual who appropriately shares information that can be used in many different and morally acceptable ways cannot be considered morally responsible for a later abortion anymore than the scientist who did the original genetic research.

Genetic Testing for
Children and Adolescents

A family that is at risk for a particular genetic condition might be interested in having a child tested for the mutation underlying that condition. If the test is performed to make or confirm a medical diagnosis, then it falls under general principles governing medical care. But if the test involves a late onset disease, such as Huntington's, or a predisposition to a disease, such as breast or colon cancer, then the decision is more problematic.

Parents may consider presymptomatic testing of a child for a variety of reasons: to gain peace of mind, as a basis for educational or career decisions, to identify early preventive or therapeutic interventions, or as a guide for eventual marital and reproductive choices, among other reasons. When children become aware of genetic conditions in their family, they, too, may express an interest in testing, and adolescents in particular may wish to make their own decisions about being tested.

A 2005 study by Rony Duncan of the Medical Ethics Unit of Imperial College in London found that many young people who were at risk for a genetic disease simply assumed that they would develop the disease. In a sense, these adolescents put their lives on hold, or in Duncan's words, "held their breath" until they were able to be tested. Duncan concluded that for many of these young people, who had to wait until they were adults to consent to testing, an earlier test would have been beneficial.

Professional medical and genetic organizations, however, consistently oppose predictive or predispositional testing unless there is a direct and timely medical benefit to the child, such as a proven treatment or preventive strategy. Since many at-risk adults choose not to be tested, a child who is unable to make a mature and informed decision should not be subjected to a test whose results cannot be undone once the test has been performed. For some adolescents, the psychosocial benefits of testing could justify testing, but professional pretest counseling is essential in order to assess the maturity level and motivation of the individual adolescent. In addition, posttest counseling should be available to help the young person deal with test results.

Reproductive and Marital Decisions

The principles of human dignity, relationality, and solidarity described above, as well as the fundamental concept of responsible choice, apply directly to consideration of reproductive and marital decisions related to genetic testing.

Preventing the Transmission of Genetic Diseases
The healing mission supported by the Catholic Church recognizes that preventing a disease or disabling condition is generally preferable to trying to deal with its effects later on. Prospective parents hope for the birth of a healthy child, and obstetric providers make preconception and prenatal recommendations in hopes of achieving this aim. The goal is not perfectionism but the basic health status that is the foundation for normal human flourishing.

The Church has specifically recognized this goal, since one of the impediments to valid marriage—blood relationship—was originally linked to the belief that the offspring of two closely related individuals were at risk of physical and mental disorders. Blood relationship was used to identify couples who were likely to transmit a hereditary defect, thus implying that the prevention of such diseases was regarded as desirable by the Church.

Responsible Parenthood

Because of advances in genomics, we now know much more about the transmission of hereditary disease and reproductive decisions have become more complex. The concept of *responsible parenthood*, expounded by the bishops of Vatican Council II in their *Pastoral Constitution on the Church in the Modern World*, provides guidance for reproductive decisions. Couples are advised to consider five criteria:

(1) The good of the marriage
(2) The good of the children, those born and those yet to come
(3) Financial and other resources
(4) Spiritual development
(5) The good of the Church and society

Some, if not all, of these criteria are affected by information about genetic conditions and risks for transmitting genetic diseases. The principle of relationality is expressed prominently in three of the criteria: the good of the marriage, the good of all the children, and the good of the larger community. Responsible parenthood requires consideration of all these relationships when reproductive decisions are made.

The bishops' instruction also noted that a reproductive decision is a personal and individual decision, to be made by the couple themselves. It is not appropriate for medical professionals to identify the "right" decision, or for counselors to advise a particular choice. Conversely, a couple faced with a difficult reproductive decision should not transfer responsibility for their decision to a physician or counselor.

When it comes to genetic risks among Catholics, responsible parenthood may lead to a decision not to have biological children, or additional biological children, perhaps accompanied by the choice of adoption. In a 1951 "Address to Midwives," Pope Pius XII explicitly supported a couple's decision to prevent the conception of severely diseased offspring through avoiding intercourse during the woman's fertile period "even for the entire duration of the marriage."

If carrier testing were done prior to marriage, it could result in a decision by two carriers of the same mutation not to marry. Alternatively, a couple might decide that they are able to accept the prospect of a genetically compromised child, even though the decision could create certain burdens. Many options are permissible within Catholic teaching, and each couple must make their own decision based on the criteria for responsible parenthood.

Prenatal Diagnosis

Prenatal diagnosis is often assumed to be useful only for a couple that intends to terminate a pregnancy if the test results indicate a genetic or chromosomal disorder. This assumption is incorrect, as some couples wish to have advance warning of a disease or disabling condition so they can make preparations. Preparations might include concrete plans such as delivery at a site equipped to care for the newborn, as well as the parents' own psychological and emotional readiness.

Prenatal testing services offered by Catholic and other pro-life organizations can offer a safe context for potential parents who might feel pressure from other providers to terminate a pregnancy in response to positive test results. Such organizations can offer support for a couple's decision to continue the pregnancy, and should also assist a couple that gives birth to a disabled or sick child to obtain resources and assistance in caring for that child's medical and developmental needs.

Before choosing to have prenatal diagnosis through amniocentesis, however, a couple needs to understand that the procedure itself presents some risk to the pregnancy. If their purpose in requesting the procedure is solely for reassurance, then they will want to examine whether this benefit outweighs the risk. In any case, the risk of miscarriage or other harm to the fetus is not acceptable unless there is a specific reason for testing, such as family history or advanced maternal age. For appropriate patients, the availability of noninvasive screening for some disorders offers a great advantage in avoiding the risks of amniocentesis.

Carrier Screening

Until recently, only persons who had a family history of a genetic disorder and their reproductive partners were screened for carrier status in relation to that specific disorder. However, in 1997 a conference at the National Institutes of Health recommended that cystic fibrosis (CF) carrier screening be expanded to all couples planning a pregnancy or seeking prenatal care. This recommendation was implemented in 2001 through guidelines developed by the American College of Obstetricians and Gynecologists in collaboration with the American College of Medical Genetics.

When screened during an ongoing pregnancy, if a couple found they were both CF carriers, they would have to decide whether to proceed with prenatal diagnosis for a fetus that had a 25 percent probability of having cystic fibrosis. For a couple at the stage of planning a pregnancy, positive test results would allow them to consider other options. They could decide not to take the risk involved in becoming pregnant. They might be advised to consider preimplantation genetic diagnosis (PGD) in conjunction with in vitro fertilization. However, this procedure is not acceptable under Catholic teaching since it involves genetic diagnosis of embryos followed by the discarding of affected embryos two or three days after fertilization.

The guidelines for CF-carrier screening emphasize the importance of adequate information and fully informed consent by the couple before testing is performed. No one is required to accept carrier screening. In addition, the guidelines reinforce the responsibility of patients with positive tests to inform relatives that they are also at risk. Materials provided include a sample letter that a patient could send to family members and relatives. This sample letter accomplishes three goals. It implies that notification of relatives is normal or expected, it ensures that information about the meaning of carrier status is accurate, and it makes notification physically (if not psychologically) easy.

Premarriage Screening

If carrier screening (such as CF screening) is now recommended for couples planning a pregnancy, could it also be offered to couples as part of premarriage preparation? What about screening for other disorders for which particular couples may be at risk?

As noted earlier, the main tool for identifying hereditary conditions for which an individual may be at risk is the family history. Family history forms could be included in marriage preparation packets for all couples marrying in a Catholic church. The family history might identify couples who could benefit from professional genetic counseling, possibly leading to genetic testing for a specific condition.

But the main purpose of the forms would be to encourage couples to discuss what they would do if certain types of situations arose. Did they agree or disagree, for example, on the acceptability of abortion in case of fetal defect? If the prospective spouses found that they disagreed significantly on how they would want to handle potential reproductive decisions, they might want to reconsider their marriage plans.

Pharmacogenomics

In the near future, genomics and genetic testing may have their greatest impact in relation to the prescription of medications and new drug development. For example, drug studies suggest that patients respond differently to drugs that are prescribed to lower their blood pressures or cholesterol levels, and at least part of this difference may be attributable to variations in genetic makeup. Therefore, genetic testing may eventually help physicians prescribe the drug that will be most effective for a particular patient rather than relying on a trial-and-error approach. Knowledge of a patient's genetic makeup can also help avoid adverse reactions to a particular drug or regulate the appropriate dosage, as has recently been shown for the blood-thinning drug Warfarin.

In the area of drug development, research may show that a drug that is not demonstrably effective for the target population as a whole may have a positive response in a subset of the population with a particular genetic characteristic. Thus, rather than being abandoned, the drug may be tested on that subset of patients and may prove effective and even lifesaving for them. Drug companies, however, are not likely to find it profitable to develop and test drugs that would be used by only a small number of patients. This challenge can sometimes be overcome through incentives or through grants and research conducted by public agencies that are not so dependent on profit in the marketplace.

Questions for Discussion

1. Under what circumstances would it be appropriate for adults to seek genetic testing? What about children and adolescents?
2. If you had to make a decision to undergo genetic testing, what factors would go into making that decision?

3. Do you think that genetics should enter into decisions about getting married? Should genetic science influence the decision to have children?

4. Do you agree that the information that results from genetic testing is not the exclusive property of the individual, but may at times have to be shared with family members? Explain.

5. What do you see as strengths and weaknesses of genetic testing?

For Further Reading

Atkinson, Gary M., and Albert S. Moraczewski. *Genetic Counseling, the Church, & the Law.* St. Louis, Mo.: Pope John XXIII Medical-Moral Research and Education Center, 1980.

Hamel, Ronald P., and Michael R. Panicola. "What's a Catholic to Think? A Genomics That Promotes Human Flourishing Can Extend Jesus' Mission." *Health Progress* Volume 85 (May–June 2004): 23–26.

O'Rourke, Kevin D., and Philip Boyle, eds. *Medical Ethics: Sources of Catholic Teachings,* third ed. Washington, DC: Georgetown University Press, 1999.

Shannon, Thomas A., and James J. Walter. *The New Genetic Medicine: Theological and Ethical Reflections.* Lanham, Md.: Rowman & Littlefield Publishers, 2003.

Smith, David H., and Cynthia B. Cohen, eds. *A Christian Response to the New Genetics: Religious, Ethical, and Social Issues.* Lanham, Md.: Rowman & Littlefield Publishers, 2003.

Smith, David H., et al. *Early Warning: Cases and Ethical Guidance for Presymptomatic Testing in Genetic Diseases.* Bloomington Ind.: Indiana University Press, 1998.

CHAPTER **3**

Making Decisions about Organ Transplantation

Patricia A. Talone, RSM, PhD

WW ere it not for the generosity of strangers," Diane mused, "I
wouldn't be here to enjoy life or to give back some of what
God has given me." Diane is not her real name, but her story is true
and reflects that of countless other organ recipients. Over fifteen
years ago, shortly after she had completed her master's degree in
liturgical music and while actively involved in a large, suburban
parish, Diane began to be troubled by headaches and high blood
pressure. These symptoms were eventually diagnosed as a rare form
of kidney disease. Nothing she tried was able to halt the deterioration of her kidney function, and she soon had to rely upon triweekly
dialysis. Diane's doctors put her name on an organ donation waiting list, as she, her family, and numerous friends prayed for a lifesaving match. After almost a year, the call came, and she received
the kidney of a middle-aged woman who had died from a brain
aneurysm. Diane's donor's family, desirous to share the gift of their
loved one's life with others, were able to provide organs to five persons who otherwise would have died or experienced severe physical
limitations. Diane has come to a deeper understanding of the meaning of an individual or family offering a vital part of their bodies.

"For me," she says, "this total, unselfish gift enhances the Catholic eucharistic understanding of Jesus' self-donation so that others might live."

How did the donor family decide to give these final gifts? Was theirs a strictly altruistic impulse, a desire to make the best of a truly tragic loss? Did this wife and mother leave written instructions regarding her wishes to donate? Were they guided by their religious beliefs? Diane doesn't know the answer to these questions, but expresses her gratitude to God for her donor and the donor's family each day of her life. She occasionally speaks at civic and parish meetings, encouraging others to think about the possibility of donating a vital organ, bone marrow, or tissue. She urges them to talk with their loved ones, and to put instructions in writing so as not to leave loved ones to face a very difficult decision at an emotionally stressful time.

It is hard to believe that the treatment choices and decisions many individuals currently face were not even dreamed about prior to the first human kidney transplant in 1954. As medical miracles have become everyday reality, physicians, nurses, attorneys, legislators, and ordinary citizens have struggled to understand the very real ethical challenges that may become part and parcel of the organ donation process. While not giving definitive answers to every question donors and their families may face, Catholic teaching provides solid principles—including a rich, time-tested tradition—and spiritual guidance for physicians, patients, and families as they face these challenging questions.

Reality of the Need

As recently as the 1960s, organ transplantation was considered high-tech and experimental. Today, medical science has advanced so that transplantation is now considered therapeutic. While organ donation rates have slowly increased, expanded criteria for admissibility to transplant programs now means that waiting lists are still growing, and the demand for organs far exceeds the availability of donors. Many avow that the demand for transplant organs in the United States has reached a critical level. The Organ Procurement and Transplantation Network (OPTN) estimates that there are currently over eighty-nine thousand potential organ candidates on waiting lists, while the United Network for Organ Sharing (UNOS) calculates that every day, seventeen people die waiting for a vital organ. The National Kidney Foundation's Web site states that while an estimated twelve thousand persons who die in the United States each year meet the criteria for organ donation, less than half of that number actually becomes organ donors. The President's Ethics Council called the organ shortage a "tragedy for those individuals and families that wait for organs and often die waiting."

Despite the tremendous need for organs, organ donation, retrieval, and distribution remains uneven throughout the United States. According to the Joint Commission on Accreditation of Healthcare Organizations, 80 percent of organ donations are from 20 percent of all hospitals. Many of these facilities are urban, tertiary care hospitals offering state-of-the-art medical care. Just as there are disparities of medical care between ethnic and racial groups, so too, inequities exist in both donations and reception of organs for minorities. Although African Americans represent 12 percent of the overall United States population, they represent more than 35 percent of persons awaiting a kidney donation, often waiting longer than their Caucasian counterparts. These disparities evoke concern and even dismay among health care professionals, particularly so in Catholic health care, because it commits itself to reaching out to all persons, most especially those who are poor and vulnerable.

Church Teaching

Even a superficial reading of the gospels convinces one that a primary ministry during Jesus' life on earth was healing the sick and bringing comfort to those who were suffering. Often, families of the sick had all but given up hope when Jesus reached out and touched their loved one, restoring them to health. Peter's mother-in-law, Jairus's daughter, persons who were blind, lame, and leprous, all received a second chance at life through Jesus' power and intervention. Health care professionals today, whether in Catholic health care or other community and teaching hospitals throughout the country, continue Jesus' compassionate ministry to those who are sick. Organ donations are one vital aspect of continuing that mission.

Because life is a gift from a loving Creator, the sanctity of each human life has always been revered within Catholic teaching. Recognizing that human life is the highest earthly good, without which we cannot enjoy any other goods, the Catholic tradition urges us to careful stewardship for our bodies. Individuals seeking guidance when trying to decide about donation of organs and tissues need look no further than papal teaching from Pope Pius XII in the 1950s up to the addresses and writings of the late Pope John Paul II. Addressing the International Congress of Transplantation Society in August 2000, Pope John Paul II described the practice of organ donation as "a genuine act of love." In his 1995 encyclical, *Evangelium Vitae,* he maintained that "*the Gospel of life* is to be celebrated above all in *daily living* which should be filled with self-giving love for others....A particularly praiseworthy example of such gestures is the donation of organs, performed in an ethically acceptable manner, with a view to offering a chance of health and even of life itself to the sick who sometimes have no other hope" (86).

The Catholic Health Association of Canada in its *Health Ethics Guide* (2000) observes that Christians value organ and tissue donation for three reasons. First, it is an expression of the respect and dignity of every human person, and of the sanctity of each human life. Second, donation is an expression of solidarity with other members of the human community (particularly the sick, the needy, and the vulnerable). Third, donation is a call to respond in charity to the sufferings of others. In a world that increasingly succumbs to what Pope John Paul II often spoke of as "a culture of death," organ and tissue donation offers believers the opportunity to support human life by giving a part of themselves precisely so that others might live. In a June 1991 address to a congress on organ transplants, John Paul II highlighted the fact that the noble gesture of donation is based on a decision of great ethical import: "The decision to offer without reward a part of one's own body for the health and well-being of another person."

The *Catechism of the Catholic Church*, echoing the words of John Paul II, defines organ donation as a concrete sign of solidarity and self-giving love (see 2301). Similarly, the United States Conference of Catholic Bishops in their *Ethical and Religious Directives for Catholic Health Care Services* (2001) maintain that "Catholic health care institutions should encourage and provide the means whereby those who wish to do so may arrange for the donation of their organs and bodily tissue" (63). Catholic medical ethics principles, developed over many centuries, always reflecting upon new medical progress, encourage participation in scientific and technological advances while offering caution, critique, and guidance for the faithful. We will next examine some commonly discussed issues regarding organ donation and transplantation in light of Catholic teaching.

Two Types of Organ Donation
Cadaveric (sudden death) Donation

Transplanting tissue or organs from a dead person to a living person presents no ethical problems. Pope Pius XII, in a 1956 address to a group of eye specialists, spoke about such donations noting that

> A person may will to dispose of his [sic] body and to destine it to ends that are useful, morally irreproachable and even noble, among them the desire to aid the sick and suffering. One may make a decision of this nature with respect to his own body with full realization of the reverence which is due it...this decision should not be condemned but positively justified.

The Canadian Catholic Health Association sets forth clear principles to guide organ and tissue donation when the donor is dead. First, vital organs that occur singly in the body (that is, there is only one such organ, for example, the heart) may only be removed after the death of the donor. Second, the donor's consent should be well informed and freely given in advance. If the consent has not been given prior to death, either in writing or in discussion, then the consent of the family or surrogate is needed. Third, there must be moral certainty that the donor is, in fact, dead. The donor must be pronounced dead by a physician.

In general, the American public understands that organs may be donated from someone who has recently died. Many states distribute organ donation cards or forms on a regular basis. While this attempt to reach a broad segment of the population is laudable, often persons who fill out donor cards do not discuss their wishes with their families. Families must then come to a difficult decision at a time of tremendous emotional anguish and stress.

Living Donation

Organ donation between living persons has now surpassed that of deceased donations, primarily due to living kidney donation, which represents 94 percent of all living donations. The first living organ donation was performed between twenty-three-year-old identical twins in 1954 in Boston. Since then, thousands of patients have received such donations. In addition to kidneys, healthy persons can donate segments of the liver, lung, or pancreas. There are several reasons why living organ donation may be an advantage over cadaveric donation. First, it reduces the wait time for the recipient (thus minimizing the risks of further physical deterioration). Second, it permits surgery to be scheduled ahead of time, adequately preparing the surgical staff as well as patients and family for the serious surgery. Third, it reduces the cold-ischemia time, that is, the time that the vital organ is stored without oxygenated blood.

There are three categories of donation by living persons. First among these is *directed donation* to a loved one or a friend. Often a parent or sibling may donate an organ or part of an organ to a relative in need. The second type is *non-directed donation*. In this case, the donor gives an organ to the general pool to be transplanted into the recipient in greatest need. The third type is *directed donation to a stranger*, in which donors choose to give to a specific person with whom they have no prior social or emotional connection. The second and third type are sometimes called *altruistic donation*.

More ethical quandaries may arise in organ donation between living persons than with dead donors. For example, how can one determine when the need outweighs the risk of undergoing unnecessary (nontherapeutic) surgery in order to donate an organ to a family member, or even a complete stranger? Would one possibly jeopardize one's own life and violate the principle of stewardship for their own body? According to Robert Truog, MD (*The New England Journal of Medicine*, August 4, 2005), each category of living donation carries with it ethical concerns. With directed donation to a loved one, the concern could be pressure to donate, or coercion. A parent might feel that he or she must donate to save a dying child. In the informed consent process, physicians must prevent donors from taking life-threatening risks for reasons that do not proportionately justify the risk. Both nondirected and directed donation to a stranger demands that transplant teams carefully scrutinize the donor. They must insure that an altruistic donation is based on sound psychological reasons and informed consent. Truog even cautions that some altruistic donations could evolve into a slippery slope toward the buying and selling of organs.

While ethicists have discussed the implications of these transplants since the 1940s, there has not been unanimity about the principle that would justify such a donation. Catholic medical ethicists in the first third of the twentieth century taught that one should not undergo surgery that was not therapeutic. Thus, unnecessary surgeries for purely cosmetic purposes, for example, were clearly frowned upon. The principle of stewardship of the body demanded that an individual should not in any way threaten or harm the health and integrity of his or her body. Jesuit moral theologian, Gerald Kelly, on the other hand, allowed for living donations under what he called "the principle of fraternal love," provided there was only limited harm to the donor. Other Catholic ethicists, notably Charles J. McFadden in his 1976 book, *The Dignity of Life: Moral Values in a Changing Society*, distinguished between strict anatomical integrity and functional integrity. The former he described as the physical integrity of the body, while the latter is the systematic efficiency of the body. A classic example of this distinction would be an individual who is born with only one kidney. He or she might lack anatomical integrity, but maintains functional integrity, with the single kidney purifying the entire body.

The Ethical and Religious Directives for Catholic Health Care

Respect for human dignity on the part of the health care professional demands that he or she should not ask a patient to undergo any medical treatment or procedure without first obtaining the patient's informed consent from either the patient or surrogate. This means that the health professional (usually one's primary care physician or surgeon, but sometimes a physician assistant or nurse practitioner) must take the time to discuss with the individual the benefits and burdens of the proposed treatment, possible alternatives, and any possible side effects or consequences. In today's fast-paced medical environment, some physicians and nurses give the patient a printed brochure containing pertinent medical information. Federal law requires that patients must sign a consent form before undergoing any surgery or receiving treatment. However, signing a form or reading a pamphlet does not necessarily mean that one has received or given fully informed consent.

Just as it is incumbent upon the physician to discuss the proposed surgery with a patient, and to probe to ascertain whether the patient fully understands the procedure, so too, the responsible patient must carefully read the materials he or she receives. It is good to write down questions that one might have before visiting the doctor's office, since one can easily forget even vital questions in a hurried or stressful environment. It is always better to ask questions before giving consent than to have second thoughts after one has already granted permission.

Most living donations are given from a relative of the recipient. While even this type of donation is not without its challenges, some in the transplant community express concern regarding what are called altruistic donations. These are donations made from individuals who may not even know the recipient, but who learn of their need through the media, friends, and so on. Catholic teaching tells us that true charity, or *agape*, is indeed a valid motive for donation, but ethicists and organ procurement organizations (OPO) warn that extra protections may be needed to ensure that this is truly a free donation. For the most part, living donors are asked to undergo a psychosocial evaluation to protect both the donor and the recipient. OPOs insist that consent for altruistic donation be more voluntary and less unduly influenced than that between related donors and recipients.

Buying and Selling of Organs

Despite the fact that the Organ Transplantation Act of 1984 prohibits the buying and selling of organs as well as direct compensation to a living donor or a deceased donor's family, organ markets exist throughout the world. In some cases, donors are paid for organs and the recipients pay for them, creating a market in human organs. A casual perusal of the Internet reveals sites dedicated to ending the organ shortage by allowing monetary compensation for cadaveric organs, which, they say, will greatly increase the current low supply. One site proposes compensation for cadaveric organs only, but others encourage living persons to sell kidneys and portions of livers. While the goal of "increasing organ supply" might be laudable, one is left wondering if the reason for this encouragement arises from altruism and love of neighbor, to provide money to a cash-strapped donor, or to increase "business" for transplant surgeons and centers.

On a public policy level, the President's Council, a committee consisting of physicians, philosophers, and others, in 2003 rejected such exchanges, acknowledging the tragic reality that "by setting moral limits and outlawing 'cash for flesh,' we may be decreasing organ supply—and thus accepting the suffering and death of those we might have saved, at least temporarily." The Council cautioned that in setting aside moral limits or treating the human body and its parts as property, even with the hope of increasing the organ supply and saving lives, our society would run the risk of devaluing the very human life and human bodies that we seek to save.

Pope John Paul II, in his August 29, 2000, address, likewise rejected "any procedure which tends to commercialize" human organs or consider them items of exchange or trade because to use the body as an object is to fundamentally violate the dignity of the human person. He based this censure on the fact that organ donation is not giving away something that belongs to us (property), but giving something of our very selves. The human body, he argues, is not simply a complex of tissue and organs, but a constitutive part of the person.

That being said, within the medical transplant community, conversations persist about incentives for deceased donation. Recognizing that the need for organs often disproportionately affects the poor and persons of color, Pennsylvania legislators proposed indirect incentives to the families of donors by suggesting that the family could receive financial assistance for the donor's funeral. Other incentives proposed include tax breaks for living donation and what is termed "directed donation." The latter proposes to give priority to donors on organ waiting lists, should this individual later be in need of a transplant. While debate about financial assistance for donor families may continue, there is general consensus within the ethical and transplant communities that selling organs is unethical.

Definition of Death

Because we so reverence the dignity of each and every human life, we can never remove vital organs until after the donor has died. Although this requirement might seem self-evident, John Paul II has pointed out that "to act otherwise would mean intentionally to cause the death of the donor in disposing of his [sic] organs" (August

20, 2000). How, then, does one define death? The U.S. Uniform
Determination of Death Act of 1983 (UDDA) stated that death may
be declared when a person sustains either (1) irreversible cessation
of circulatory and respiratory functions, or (2) irreversible cessation of all functions of the entire brain, including the brain stem.
These two ways of ascertaining death are otherwise known as cardio-
respiratory (heart and lungs) death, and brain death.

At a 2005 National Conference on Donation After Cardiac
Death, over two hundred physicians, medical policy experts, and
ethicists worked together to clarify definitions and propose careful
guidelines for medical protocols. Building upon the UDDA, the
group confirmed that the diagnosis of death requires (1) cessation
of functions and (2) irreversibility. Cessation of functions is recognized by an appropriate clinical examination that reveals the absence of responsiveness, heart sounds, pulse, and respiratory effort.
In other words, the patient's heart and breathing have stopped. Irreversibility is recognized by persistent cessation of function during an appropriate period of observation. The group recognized
that individual health care facility protocols will determine exactly
how long this "appropriate period" might be. It did note that "when
life sustaining therapy is withdrawn, based on the limited data available, spontaneous circulation does not return after two minutes of
cessation of circulation." While some facilities require a ten-minute
wait after CR cessation, most required a five-minute wait. It is important to note that laws governing organ donation insist that the
physician making the declaration of death may not be one connected
with the organ transplant team. Such safeguards ensure the public
trust in the organ donation process and prevent any conflict of interests for health care professionals involved.

Donation after Cardiac Death

Most cadaveric organ donors die from a traumatic head injury, often caused by an accident like a car crash or a fall. Physicians may declare the individual brain dead even though his or her heart and lungs continue to function because the patient remains on a ventilator. However, most persons do not die from head injuries, but from other illnesses, and therefore cannot become organ donors after death, even though they might have indicated they wished to do so. In the past few years, following the guidelines of the Institute of Medicine (2000), many states have initiated organ protocols called Non-Heart-Beating Organ Donation (NHBD) or, more recently, Donation after Cardiac Death (DCD). In these protocols, death must be declared within a few minutes after cardio-respiratory functions cease. If physicians wait too long after declaring death before removing the organs, the delay damages solid organs because of lack of blood flow and oxygen throughout the body.

For the most part, these donors—patients who are on life support—have no real chance of survival and, as such, their families or surrogates decide to withdraw life support. The family and medical staff recognize that the patient is dying, and will probably die quickly once life-sustaining treatment is removed. It is possible for families to request organ donation and to provide for an organ transplant team to arrive before removal of life support. Again, safety measures ensure respect for both the donor and the recipient, prevent conflicts of interests, and ensure the fiduciary responsibility of the professionals and the health care institution.

Many DCD protocols require that physicians administer a large dose of the drug heparin after life support has begun to be withdrawn, but before death is declared. Heparin is an anticoagulant used to maintain a proper blood flow in newly procured organs so that they can be better preserved for the transplantation. Some ethicists (for example, Peter Clark and Uday Deshmukh in *The National Catholic Bioethics Quarterly*, Autumn 2004) contend that heparin is contraindicated in patients with bleeding or head injuries. In these cases, they argue that an anticoagulant could cause more severe bleeding and thus directly (rather than indirectly) cause death. Others, like James DuBois, believe that heparin is good at preventing clots but not quickly dissolving them. He argues that one can apply the principle of double effect to the use of heparin for DCD because: (1) the medication has a legitimate purpose and is not evil in itself; (2) the risk of causing death is foreseen but not intended; (3) the risk of hemorrhage is not a means to the end of thinning the blood for transplant; and (4) if the patient is in the process of dying, it may be consistent with the patient's wishes, and thus proportionate.

While ethicists and physicians will continue to discuss the efficacy and morality of the use of heparin, families and surrogates should heed the advice of the Institute of Medicine. It counsels that decisions regarding drugs should be made on a case-by-case basis. Transplant teams should obtain informed consent from families regarding the use of any medication that does not directly benefit the donor. While the transplant community is rightly committed to increasing the number of potentially transplantable organs, the responsibility of surrogates is to make the best decision for the donor.

Conclusion

Transplants, Pope John Paul II maintained, are a great step forward in science's service of humankind, and many today owe their lives to an organ transplant. "Increasingly, the technique of transplants has proven to be a valid means of attaining the primary goal of all medicine—the service of human life" (August 29, 2000). Just as Diane thanks God every day for her gift of renewed life, so, too, do countless women and men who selflessly offered the gift of life to others by donating the organs of their loved ones. Gratitude and hope fill their hearts.

Ask Mary and Bill, a couple who generously donated the organs of their oldest son, Steven. Steve was a faith-filled, energetic, enthusiastic nineteen-year-old when he was tragically struck down in a bicycle accident. Keeping vigil at his bedside, Mary recalled that her son had indicated on his license that he wanted to donate his organs so that others might live. Besides having guidance from their now brain-dead son, Mary recalls their firm conviction that they did not want any other parents or siblings to lose their loved ones. If Steve's organs could help others to live, they would be fulfilling their faith commitment to share the gift of life that God had so generously bestowed upon him. Steve's heart, kidneys, liver, corneas, and bone tissue were successfully transplanted. This devout Catholic couple fulfilled Pope John Paul's call to "nurture a culture of life" through their compassion, generosity, and hope. Not a day goes by, Mary says, that she does not recall with both joy and sadness their beloved son. But her pain is accompanied by a deep sense of comfort in this "genuine act of love."

Questions for Discussion

1. Have you made provisions to donate your organs after your death? Why? Why not?
2. What, if any, concerns do you have about organ donation in any of its forms?
3. What is your view of selling organs or of a donor or donor family being compensated for a donation?
4. What ethical guidance does this chapter provide for making decisions about organ donation?

For Further Reading

Clark, Peter and Uday Deshmukh. "Non-Heart-Beating Organ Donation and Catholic Ethics." *The National Catholic Bioethics Quarterly.*
Autumn 2004, 537–551.

Cox, Johnny and Carol Bayley. "Organ Donation and Prudential
Deliberation." *Health Progress,* January–February 2001, 22–24.

DuBois, James. "Non-Heart-Beating Organ Donation." *Health Progress,*
January–February, 2001, 18–21.

Pope John Paul II. "Address to the 18th International Congress of the
Transplantation Society." August 29, 2000.

National Catholic Bioethics Center. "Giving Something of Ourselves."
Ethics and Medics. August 2002. Issue reprints relevant sections from
The Catholic Organizations for Life and Family (Canada) and the
Catholic Health Association of Canada, as well as sections from the
Catechism of the Catholic Church.

Truog, Robert. "The Ethics of Organ Donation by Living Donors." *The
New England Journal of Medicine,* August 4, 2005.

CHAPTER **4**

Making Decisions about End-of-Life Care

Richard C. Sparks, CSSP, PhD

A nyone who has lived as a Catholic the last twenty to thirty years surely knows that our Church is "pro-life." Pope John Paul II spent much of his papacy preaching and teaching about respecting human life from the moment of conception to the time of one's natural death. We're a Church that is strongly antiabortion, increasingly critical of the death penalty, and that promotes peace, not war. Jesus says, "I came that they may have life, and have it abundantly" (John 10:10).

Some Catholics, however, misinterpret our pro-life stance to mean primarily life-in-the-body or life-here-on-earth. But Jesus proclaims a view of life that is both *earthly* and *eternal*, here as well as beyond the grave. "I am the resurrection and the life," he says. "Those who believe in me, even though they die, will live, and everyone who lives and believes in me will never die" (John 11:25–26).

In the United States the late Cardinal Joseph Bernardin of Chicago, for many years chair of the Bishops' Pro-Life Committee, synthesized much of this holistic respect-for-life in what he called "a consistent ethic of life," viewing all life issues together as "a seamless garment." Pope John Paul II gave further shape to this underlying Catholic pro-life belief in his 1995 encyclical *The Gospel of Life (Evangelium vitae)*. Speaking clearly about life in its various stages, the pope declared: "It is in being destined to life in its fullness, to "eternal life," that many person's earthly life acquires its full meaning" (*EV*, 80).

Thus Catholic teaching across the centuries has consistently said that, as natural death draws near, it is not necessary and may even be futile to fight it at all costs.

Illness, aging, and finally death-of-the-body are a natural part of the life cycle for us all. As they say somewhat humorously, "No one gets out of this life alive," at least not "alive" in an earthly or bodily sense. Death is the inevitable and natural last stage of earthly life, opening us up to the fullness of eternal life.

So, to "respect life" means to make decisions that enhance our lives *as a whole*. Throughout most of our lives, the obvious medical decision is to "forge ahead"—take your medicine, undergo the surgery, do the prescribed treatment that will save your life and enhance your health. But at some point, forestalling the inevitable onset of dying may be futile, wasteful, torturous, and morally wrong.

At any given juncture in life we are called to make "the right decision" for this time, this place, this circumstance. "But that sounds like relativism or *situation ethics*," some might say. No, it merely means that the Catholic moral tradition—rooted in the gospels, the writings of great theologians like Augustine and Aquinas, and the life experience of Catholic people and pastors across the centuries— is realistic and circumstantial, applying timeless values to historical situations.

This chapter focuses on making good, life-respecting end-of-life decisions. Death may not be imminent. It might be a question of how best to live our lives here and now, even when death is not foreseen: With or without a painful, costly, and risky surgery? With or without a proposed chemotherapy regimen? On dialysis or not? At home or in a long-term care facility?

The Catholic medical ethics tradition concerning these "to treat" or "not to treat" decisions is a rich resource. Rooted in Scripture and Tradition, we find its first full expression in the 1500s. Spanish scholars of the Counter-Reformation era (for example, Francisco de Vitoria, Domingo Soto, Domingo Bañez) crafted language that many of us today know as "ordinary" versus "extraordinary" means. Most Catholics have some intuition that if a proposed therapy is "ordinary," we should use it; if "extraordinary" it would not be morally required. This concept, vital in the Catholic moral tradition, is a helpful tool for health care decisions.

So let's use this helpful piece of our Catholic heritage as we try to respond to some of the following questions: (1) Who decides? (2) When, if ever, is it morally right to say, "Halt—No more treatments"? Another way of saying this might be, "On what basis is it moral to stop or forego further medical efforts to save a patient's life?" (3) If nontreatment is the decision, what's next? What, in terms of basic hygienic and nursing care, is mandatory? (4) Is it ever permissible to forego or disconnect tube feeding? (5) What about alleviating pain and suffering for a dying person? When, if ever, are we justified to use morphine or other narcotics to ease the pain of dying patients or those in severe discomfort? Is this a form of euthanasia or simply humane medical care? (6) And finally, given the legalization of physician-assisted suicide in Oregon and euthanasia in the Netherlands, is it ever *morally* justified to assist a dying patient to end his/her life (that is, assisted suicide)?

Who Decides?
Who Should Make Medical
Decisions for You?

The Catholic answer parallels that adopted by most of Western ethics and medicine. Who decides? Ideally the competent patient decides for himself or herself. Hospitals use the language of *autonomy*, *privacy*, and *informed consent* to express this priority given to the patient's own wishes. One might better respond to the "who decides" question by saying: Ideally the competent patient decides, but not in isolation. It is up to the physician and health care professionals to inform the patient reasonably well: diagnosis, treatment options, insurance coverage, costs, benefits, burdens, side effects, alternatives, and so forth. Provided the patient is alert and mentally competent enough to understand, then he or she has the right to make decisions about his or her future life.

Some have suggested that it might be better to let the doctor or some objective third party make the medical-moral judgment. But the Catholic tradition and mainstream medical ethics agree that the patient's perspective—including life goals, values, and fears—is relevant to making "the right" decision. Whether a given surgery or treatment is "worth it" is not solely a matter of its physical effects. How one perceives his or her ability to cope and live and flourish is a somewhat intangible but very real piece of the decision. So, taking into account loved ones and social responsibilities, the data and best advice of the medical team, a reasonably competent patient remains the ultimate decision maker.

Advance Directives and Living Wills

But what if I'm no longer competent? What if I'm in a coma or later stages of dementia or Alzheimer's? Who decides then? With just such cases in mind, advance directives were created. An advance directive is the generic term for any form of document in which a competent patient tries to state in advance what to do if and when he or she no longer is able to speak for himself or herself. "Living will" is the common name given to this kind of document in which a person tries to delineate in advance *what* precisely he or she would want (or not want) if and when the time comes.

The earliest versions of living wills were often brief and succinct. For example, "If I'm terminally ill and not expected to recover, I would *not* want excessive or extraordinary medical measures used to prolong my life." It seems clear and to the point. However, if, as noted above, a patient rightly may bring one's own personal life, religious faith, and values to bear in judging "excessive or extraordinary," then declaring any treatment categorically *ordinary* or *extraordinary* would seem nearly impossible. One person's excessive and extraordinary might be another person's acceptable and ordinary.

Since this early era of living wills, some have begun to craft more and more detailed documents, attempting to cover a variety of treatment options for a battery of diseases, as well as differing decisions at various stages of each disease. One physician wrote a fifty-page living will, attempting to cover all the possibilities. It's next to impossible to craft a prepackaged living will that expresses one's wishes covering any and all circumstances.

Thus a second kind of advance directive was devised. This version tells others *who* to turn to, as in: Whom do I designate as my "proxy" spokesperson? This kind of advance directive is called a "durable power of attorney for health care." It's not to be confused with the "durable power of attorney." The latter is a document giving control of one's finances should a person ever become incompetent. Whereas the former designates someone whom I trust and empowers this person to make *health care* decisions on my behalf.

It is presumed that one's designated proxy will hear the diagnosis, prognosis, and treatment options; weigh the pros and cons *according to the value system of the patient*, and make a decision. In our current culture, physicians, health care institutions, their ethics committees, and civil courts all seem to be more comfortable with this proxy option than with a hard-and-fast living will. Naming the *who*, rather than listing the *what*, seems to allow for greater situational discernment and case variations. Some folks try for the best of both options by writing a "combination document," proxy plus living will. In this hybrid form they not only designate the person (that is, the proxy) to speak in their behalf but also state at least some values and parameters to help guide the future discussion after they can no longer personally participate.

Noncompetent Patients with No Advance Directive

Finally, in the area of "who decides," there is the question of the never-competent patient (such as the *severely* brain damaged or mentally disabled) or the no-longer-competent patient (such as comatose or severe dementia). Who decides for them? If one is not competent to decide for oneself and has not left an advance directive, then it is up to the spouse, parents, family, and caregivers to arrive at a decision *in the best interest of the patient*, considered as a whole (body, mind, and spirit).

Most state laws build in a tiered approach. Usually, the wishes of the spouse of an incompetent adult patient take precedence over parents or siblings. For children, parents or legal guardians are the primary decision makers. The health care providers serve not as primary deciders, but as professional supervisors, overseeing and facilitating the decision-making process for a given family. If abuse or ulterior motives are suspected, the doctor or others may ask for a consultation from that facility's ethics committee or the civil courts.

"To Treat" or "Not to Treat"—
On What Basis Should One Decide?

In 2001, the United States Conference of Catholic Bishops issued a revised version of their official guidelines, *Ethical and Religious Directives for Catholic Health Care Services* (1995, 2001). Directives 56 and 57 answer the above question succinctly:

> A person has a moral obligation to use ordinary or proportionate means of preserving his or her life. Proportionate means are those that in the judgment of the patient offer a reasonable hope of benefit and do not entail an excessive burden or impose excessive expense on the family or the community (56).

In an attempt to clarify when treatment would *not* be required Directive 57 says:

> A person may forego extraordinary or disproportionate means of preserving life. Disproportionate means are those that in the patient's judgment do not offer a reasonable hope of benefit or entail an excessive burden, or impose excessive expense on the family or the community.

So how does one measure *reasonable* in terms of "hope of benefit" and *excessive* in terms of "burden or expense"? And how should one balance one's own benefits and burdens with those mentioned for family or the wider community? According to the official *Vatican Declaration on Euthanasia* (1980), issued by then Cardinal Joseph Ratzinger, with the approval of Pope John Paul II:

[I]t will be possible to make a correct judgment as to the means by studying the type of treatment to be used, its degrees of complexity or risk, its cost and the possibilities [availability] of using it, and comparing these elements with the results that can be expected, taking into account the state of the sick person and his or her physical and moral resources (section IV).

At this point, it may be more evident to the reader why we argue that the competent patient is the best moral decision-maker. Who knows better how all of this data will impact his or her own health and state of mind? Will the proposed therapy save my life? If so, for how long? At what level of health? Will I be mobile? Can I go home? Will I be able to work again? What about physical pain or mental suffering? Will my insurance cover the costs? If not, how will I pay the bill? What kinds of burden and inconvenience will this impose on my spouse and family? Are they able to undertake such burdens in my behalf? Is it worth it to me? To them? Or, perhaps more importantly, what will be the state of my relationships (for example, as spouse, parent, provider, Catholic, citizen, and so on)?

These are objective questions whose answers are always contextual. For example, let's look at two cases involving the use of the same medical equipment—a ventilator or respirator. If I have a lung infection and the regimen of medication prescribed is for two to three weeks, is it worth it to be put on a "breathing machine" to assist my own lung capacity? Insurance will cover it. It will be for a prescribed period of time (less than a month). While there is surely some discomfort from the ventilator, these burdens seem relatively minor. In a short time I should become accustomed to them and sedatives will help me to better cope. My prognosis is for a full recovery and a return to a full and active life. Most would agree that *in this case* the ventilator is "ordinary" or "proportionate" and thus obligatory.

However, if I am rushed to the hospital after being dredged up from an icy river, should I be hooked up to the ventilator automatically? If I have been revived, and am having trouble breathing on my own, it might be medically indicated and morally wise to "hook me up" to the ventilator *in order to do further diagnostic testing* on my physical and mental conditions. But what if, after the CT scans, MRIs, and other tests, it is found that I'm permanently comatose and not likely to ever regain the ability to breathe on my own? While we began using the ventilator in good faith, are we obliged to continue it? "No." The Catholic tradition says that I (or, in this case, my proxy) would have the right to make a decision based on a *reasonable* hope of benefits versus *excessive* burdens.

Staying alive, albeit on a respirator, is a benefit. But since life-in-the-body is not the ultimate measure of life-in-its-totality, one might say that I am mentally and socially already deceased and my body has irreversibly embarked on the dying process. Now, weighing the diagnosis, prognosis, and the burdens for all involved, it may be judged disproportionate to keep me hooked up—too much burden for too little benefit.

The longest case I've read about of someone unconscious on a ventilator is 37 years, 111 days. The cost of care for such a totally dependent patient would be astronomical. Who pays? Insurance, one's family, or the government? And while the patient would be breathing, alive in the bodily sense, if permanently unconscious would he/she be "enjoying" or benefiting personally from being kept alive "artificially"? Most people would say, "No way."

So the same respirator, which seemed ordinary and thus obligatory in the case of a modest lung infection, may be judged excessive and extraordinary in the case of a comatose, more terminal patient. Removing it is viewed as "allowing" the patient to finish the dying process. It would be inappropriate to label this removal of an extraordinary means as "euthanasia" or "murder" or "mercy-killing."

Benefits and burdens must be weighed in their proper context, in the context of the patient's own life, condition, treatment options, associated burdens, family and community network, and personal value system.

According to the centuries-old Catholic tradition, refined by recent popes, Vatican documents, Catholic health care directives, and the recent *Catechism of the Catholic Church*, competent patients (or their proxies) have the right to weigh the reasonableness of health benefits versus the burdens associated with accepting further treatment to determine what is morally mandatory and what is morally optional. The *Catechism* states that if a proposed treatment is judged "optional" and "extraordinary," its use may be deemed "over-zealous" (#2278).

The architects of Vatican II described one's conscience as that "secret and core sanctuary where one is alone with God," face to face, on holy ground. There, one is obliged to make a moral decision based on one's honest interpretation of a patient's best interest, life in all its many facets—bodily, mentally, socially, and spiritually. As Pope Pius XII phrased it as far back as 1958: "A more strict obligation would be too burdensome for most men and would render the attainment of the higher, more important good too difficult. Life, health, and all temporal activities are in fact subordinated to spiritual ends."

We Catholics are unabashedly pro-life. More often than not, saving one's life is the right moral choice. But not always, because life is a value *in context*. The Church respects and defends a patient's medical-moral decisions about health care and prolonging life in relation to one's beliefs, relational commitments, and spiritual journey—one's holistic well-being. In Church talk this holistic view of life is often referred to as a patient's "totality."

If Nontreatment of One's Illness Is the Right Decision, What's Next?

One ought never to abandon care for a seriously ill or dying patient. The *Ethical and Religious Directives* of the U.S. bishops note that "[t]he task of medicine is to care even when it cannot cure" (Part 5, Issues in Care for the Dying, Introduction). We must offer terminally ill patients and those with incurable diseases food, fluids, warmth, comfort care, pain relief where possible, and also address their psychosocial needs and their spiritual well-being. Pastoral care departments and hospice programs are among those who try to incarnate our Catholic mandate to care for the whole patient, even when cure is no longer possible.

Are Medically Administered Fluid and Nutrition *Always* Required?

The short answer is "No." Like extraordinary medical means, even these life-sustaining medical measures are not absolutely required in all cases. As the U.S. bishops' *Ethical and Religious Directives* phrase it:

> There should be a presumption in favor of providing nutrition and hydration to all patients, including patients who require medically assisted nutrition and hydration, as long as this is of sufficient benefit to outweigh the burdens involved to the patient (58).

It's worth noting that there has been a debate going on within the Catholic community—bishops, theologians, ethicists, physicians, health care experts—about when one may consider tube feedings, naso-gastric tubes, stomach tubes, and so on, to be too burdensome or of too little benefit. Obviously, these medical tools help to prolong a patient's life, keeping one's bodily functions going. The question, as with the ventilator, is "how long" and to what benefit versus burdens *for the patient?*

In some instances, the patient cannot receive the liquid without aspirating (choking) and being unable to breathe. In such cases continued use of tube feeding is medically contraindicated because it could actually suffocate the patient, directly causing death. However, there are other instances in which the nutrients can be delivered to the stomach unimpeded. In these cases (for example, the feeble elderly in nursing homes, people in latter stages of Amyotrophic Lateral Scleroisis [ALS disease], those permanently unconscious or in a persistent vegetative state [PVS]), the primary, or perhaps only, benefit to the patient is that it extends his or her physical life. Some Catholic bishops and scholars believe this is a *sufficient* benefit to override any level of burden, short of "choking." Others believe that prolonged life, by medically administered means, still must pass the excessive burden test of the "extraordinary" means criterion.

For terminally ill patients in hospice settings or those with a relatively short span of life remaining (for example, hours, weeks, or months), almost all Catholic bishops and moralists acknowledge that one is *not* obliged to hook such patients up or to continue artificially administered fluid and nutrition. Accordingly, it is not mandatory for hospice programs to connect all dying patients to medically delivered fluid and nutrition. Mother Teresa's followers do not do so and no one accuses them of being callous or immoral.

It is customary in hospice settings to offer patients sips of water, tastes of ice cream or milk shakes, ice chips, or whatever comfort "by mouth" that the patient seems to desire and benefit from. But they are not force-fed their full caloric intake. By not force-feeding them—either by mouth or by tubes—the Church does not believe we are trying to kill them nor to speed up their dying process.

It is far more accurate to say that we are "getting out of the way," not burdening a patient for too little benefit. In a sense, we are striving not to prolong their dying by not prolonging their lives during this final "dying" stage of life.

However, there is far more intra-Catholic controversy about patients who are permanently unconscious or those in a PVS. While never likely to recover conscious participation in life, these patients are not at death's door, that is, they are not imminently dying solely from their state of unconsciousness. In March 2004, a year before his own death, a very frail Pope John Paul II delivered a talk at the conclusion of a conference in Rome discussing this very topic. In his short address, the pope stated that

> the administration of water and food, even when provided by artificial means, always represents a *natural means* of preserving life, not a *medical act*. Its use, furthermore, should be considered in principle *ordinary* and *proportionate*, and as such morally obligatory insofar as and until it has attained its proper finality, which in the present case [of a PVS patient] consists in providing nourishment to the patient and alleviation of his suffering.

Some interpret this papal allocution as a major policy pronouncement, tightening the Church's traditional openness to stopping tube feeding in some, or even many, cases. Others see it as a contribution by a wise and ailing pope to the ongoing dialogue and debate about patients in the most severely compromised mental states. We all want to respect their inalienable human dignity and right to life. However, terms like "in principle" in reference to it being ordinary and proportionate and the meaning of "proper finality" in weighing providing nourishment versus alleviation of the patient's suffering are not easily defined.

Catholic bishops, clergy, theologians, ethicists, and people of good will have lined up on both sides of this "feeding tube" question in the case of PVS and other unconscious patients. At present, the official Church seems to be moving in the direction of tightening the boundaries, perhaps mandating tube-feeding for all nonconscious patients. Critics worry that the implications of such a move would threaten the whole ordinary/extraordinary means tradition, possibly mandating tube feeding for all terminally ill patients, even those in hospice and home care situations. So, in this interim period of dialogue, debate, and discernment, we must proceed with caution, care, and open minds to sound moral and pastoral advice.

Pain Medication and the Terminally Ill Patient

On this topic, the Catholic moral position is fairly unanimous and long-standing. The 1980 *Vatican Declaration on Euthanasia* clearly echoes Pope Pius XII's summary of the Catholic moral tradition on this topic: "Is the suppression of pain and consciousness by the use of narcotics…permitted by religion and the morality to the doctor and the patient (even at the approach of death and if one foresees that the use of narcotics will shorten life)?"

The document proceeds to quote and paraphrase Pius XII:

> The pope said: "If no other means exist, and if, in the given circumstances, this does not prevent the carrying out of other religious and moral duties: Yes." In this case, of course, death is in no way intended or sought even if the risk of it is reasonably taken; the intention is simply to relieve pain effectively, using for this purpose painkillers available to medicine (section III).

Those familiar with the Catholic moral tradition will recognize this as a textbook case of the application of Aquinas' "Principle of Double Effect."

What does all this mean in layperson's language? As a person's death becomes inevitable, we no longer need to worry about the potential "addictive" quality of morphine or other painkilling drugs. Our sole intention is to alleviate the physical pain and some of the mental suffering the patient may experience in the dying process. We are *not* trying to kill the patient or hasten his or her death. It has been a long-standing Catholic moral maxim that physicians are free to administer proportionately larger doses of morphine and other narcotics, as long as such incremental doses are modest and designed to overcome the patient's increasing immunity to the smaller dosage.

At some point, since the patient is dying and his or her breathing is already getting more and more shallow, the next dose of morphine may—indirectly and unintentionally—also impact the shallowness of breath. The double-effect tradition assures us that as long as our medical objective and moral intention is to keep pain under control with the smallest dosage that will do the trick, we are not morally culpable if *indirectly* and *unintentionally* the patient may breath his or her last breath a tad sooner.

Directive 61 of the U.S. bishops' *Ethical and Religious Directives* is an excellent summary of this discussion:

> Patients should be kept as free of pain as possible so that they may die comfortably and with dignity, and in the place where they wish to die....Medicines capable of alleviating or suppressing pain may be given to a dying person, even if this therapy may indirectly shorten the person's life so long as the intent is not to hasten death.

What Is the Catholic Position on Assisted Suicide and Euthanasia?

Most Catholics are aware that Church teaching consistently forbids the taking of innocent life. A person who is terminally ill or in severe pain from one's underlying disease may rightly opt to forego further medical therapies, especially if futile (not of sufficient benefit) or too burdensome. So, too, that person is free to seek pain medication and other comfort techniques to minimize or alleviate his or her suffering. For example, a person may opt to die sedated, fully unconscious, if that will be a more "peaceful" way to go. Or, if one feels that being conscious, surrounded by loved ones, able to converse, listen to music, and the like, that, too, is perfectly legitimate as a way to minimize pain and suffering, to maximize one's living while dying.

But it has been the constant tradition of the Church that one should not take the next step to do anything *directly* or consciously to end one's life or to hasten death. In this sense, "allowing one to die" is not identical with "causing one to die." In his 1995 encyclical *The Gospel of Life,* the late Pope John Paul II defined euthanasia as "an action or omission which of itself and by intention causes death, with the purpose of eliminating all suffering." Pope John Paul II labeled euthanasia or assisted suicide, however well intended, "*a grave violation of the law of God*" (65). The *Catechism of the Catholic Church* phrases it this way: "Whatever its motives and means, direct euthanasia consists in putting an end to the lives of handicapped, sick, or dying persons. It is morally unacceptable" (2277).

We cannot here enter into the societal debate about whether, in a pluralistic country, it ought to be *legal* to take one's own life, even if deemed *immoral* by some or many. The Church officially decrees that the direct taking of innocent life may never be justified, morally or legally. Further, the Church believes that the social harm set in motion by legalizing assisted suicide would far outweigh any potential benefit to freedom of conscience or tolerance of pluralism. However, that does not mean the Church is not *pastorally* sensitive in the cases of suicide or assisted suicide by the terminally ill. In recent decades the Church has softened its stance concerning the burial of suicide victims in consecrated ground. Our tendency is to diminish the moral culpability of the person, due to depression, extreme anguish, or pain. Lacking full knowledge or consent of the will, the act of taking one's own life may be objectively immoral, but the person may not be fully or even minimally culpable. Thus we prayerfully commend them to the loving arms of a compassionate God, who is full of mercy and understanding.

Conclusion

Our broad and deep medical-moral tradition is something Catholics can be proud of. In the area of end-of-life decision making, the Church has a long-standing and wise tradition. We strive to be pro-life followers of Jesus, who is our Way, Truth, and Life. In terms of end-of-life decisions, God empowers us—through the gospels and our living Church tradition—to make wise, situational, personal, morally right, life-respecting decisions.

Questions for Discussion

1. In the Catholic tradition, what does it mean to "respect life" when someone is dying?
2. According to the Catholic tradition, when is it morally permissible to withhold or withdraw treatment?
3. Have you ever encountered a decision to withhold or withdraw treatment? For what reasons was that decision made?
4. Would withholding or withdrawing a feeding tube when someone is dying be "allowing to die" or "euthanasia"? Explain.

5. Do you think that advance health care directives are a useful tool to communicate your wishes if you are no longer able to do so? Explain.

For Further Reading

Devine, Richard J. *Good Care, Painful Choices: Medical Ethics for Ordinary People*. Mahwah, N.J.: Paulist Press, 2004, 3rd ed., especially 201–244.

Christie, Dolores. *Last Rights: A Catholic Perspective on End-of-life Care*. Kansas City, Mo.: Sheed & Ward, 2003.

Kelly, David F. *Contemporary Catholic Health Care Ethics*. Washington, DC: Georgetown University Press, 2004, especially part 3, 127–228.

O'Neil, Kevin and Peter Black. *The Essential Moral Handbook*. Liguori, Mo.: Liguori Publications, 2003, 2006, especially 189–219.

O'Rourke, Kevin, ed. *A Primer for Health Care Ethics: Essays for a Pluralistic Society*. Washington, DC: Georgetown University Press, 2000, 2nd edition, especially 93–142.

Sparks, Richard C. *Contemporary Christian Morality: Real Questions, Candid Responses*. New York: Crossroad, 1996, especially questions #21–40, 28–58.

Permissions

CHAPTER 5

Making Decisions about Advance Health Care Directives

Mark Miller, C.Ss.R., Ph.D.

T he tragic case of Terri Schiavo in Florida that unfolded with unprecedented coverage over several years and into the spring of 2005 raised vital questions for many people about the kind of medical care they would find acceptable at the end of their lives. In addition, in the battle between Terri's husband, Michael, who claimed to be following her wishes to remove the feeding tube, and her parents, who claimed no such wish on Terri's part, another question arose: Who will make decisions for me if I am not able to do so?

In the last three decades of the twentieth century, a series of court cases—Karen Ann Quinlan (1976), Brother Fox (1979), Claire Conroy (1985), Nancy Cruzan (1990), and Nancy B (Canada, 1992) among them—attempted to deal with these questions. Invariably, self-determination was affirmed: The individual patient is the ultimate decision maker concerning possible treatment options.

Gradually, the roles of substitute decision makers for patients unable to make their own choices were also refined. Priority is to be given to the patient's own wishes as stated in a written advance health care directive (AHCD). The next level of priority is given to the patient's wishes as expressed to a substitute decision maker (SDM)—that is, a durable power of attorney for health care, proxy, health care agent, or surrogate decision maker. Legally, clear prior directions from a no-longer competent patient are to guide the decisions of health care providers and families.

More complex, and still not perfectly clear, is the situation of the noncompetent patient who has left no written or verbal instructions about treatment—in other words, when absolutely no preferences are known. Generally, state and provincial legislation allows some combination of next-of-kin and/or physicians to make treatment decisions based upon the "best interests" of the patient. However, great caution must be exercised in these kinds of decisions.

This chapter will concentrate on the preparation of AHCDs, primarily in written form—which could include the appointment of a surrogate decision maker and/or a stipulation of one's wishes regarding treatment at the end of life. It will also encourage conversations among family members, as this form of oral communication often enables decisions to be made in the absence of written directives.

A Brief History

AHCDs trace their origin in part to the euthanasia movement. Some people wanted their written wishes, such as to be euthanized when they are no longer competent, to be legally binding. Hence, there are Catholics who strongly opposed AHCDs on principle, even though there has never been a law in North America that allows euthanasia. The difficulty of making decisions for noncompetent patients, however, opened up the possibility of using a similar kind of document to guide treatment decisions, particularly at the end of life.

Great caution was exercised in drafting legislation in various states of the U.S. and Canadian provinces that honors individuals' written wishes about treatment options at the end of life. One can never request euthanasia or assistance in committing suicide, but, in accord with legal and moral norms regarding the acceptance or refusal of treatment options when dying, the possibility arose of assisting doctors and families in the care of loved ones through written instructions.

Because of the difficulties in writing such documents and having them followed, they have not consistently fulfilled their hoped-for promise. Poorly written directives, vague and unclear instructions, unanticipated problems, and unreceptive doctors have meant that the wishes of many patients are either not being followed or cannot be followed.

As many clinical bioethicists will attest, families often say after the death of a loved one how much easier the decision making was because the patient's wishes were clearly expressed. Accordingly, after a brief review of some of the ethical issues around the use of AHCDs, the following suggestions should enable a person to prepare a satisfactory directive to benefit family and health care providers.

Official Catholic Teaching

There is no official Church teaching about AHCDs. All official teaching is aimed at the proper care of patients according to Catholic ethical principles. One of these principles is to respect the patient's own wishes after weighing the benefits and burdens of treatment, even if the patient refuses potentially lifesaving treatment because the anticipated burdens of that treatment are deemed too great.

By extension, national bishops' conferences provide guidelines for their own countries in dealing with the question of AHCDs. The United States Conference of Catholic Bishops, for example, in their *Ethical and Religious Directives for Catholic Health Care Services* include two directives about AHCDs. I quote them in full:

> In compliance with federal law, a Catholic health care institution will make available to patients information about their rights, under the laws of their state, to make an advance directive for their medical treatment. The institution, however, will not honor an advance directive that is contrary to Catholic teaching. If the advance directive conflicts with Catholic teaching, an explanation should be provided as to why the directive cannot be honored (24).

> Each person may identify in advance a representative to make health care decisions as his or her surrogate in the event that the person loses the capacity to make health care decisions. Decisions by the designated surrogate should be faithful to Catholic moral principles and to the person's intentions and values, or if the person's intentions are unknown, to the person's best interests. In the event that an advance directive is not executed, those who are in a position to know best the patient's wishes—usually family members and loved ones—should participate in the treatment decisions for the person who has lost the capacity to make health care decisions (25).

Similarly, the Canadian Catholic Conference of Bishops has published its guidelines for Catholics in *The Health Ethics Guide* as follows:

> Advance health care directives enable a person to communicate their directions concerning the type of treatment they desire should they lose their decision-making capacity.

Persons are encouraged to discuss these directives with their family and care providers and, if appropriate, to appoint a proxy before crisis situations arise. A statement of philosophy or beliefs, when included as part of a written advance health care directive, assists family and care providers to carry out the wishes of the person receiving care (40).

A person's written or oral directives are to be respected and followed when those directives do not conflict with the mission of the organization. Advance directives which seek to clarify issues surrounding end-of-life treatment are to be discussed and carried out in a compassionate and sensitive manner (41).

One can see a certain caution in both U.S. and Canadian bishops' statements about any potential misuse of AHCDs. Nonetheless, there are currently no states or provinces that would allow euthanasia or assisted suicide in a written directive. (Oregon allows physicians to prescribe a lethal dose of drugs for assisted suicide under strict conditions, but the state does not allow the ending of the life of a noncompetent patient.)

Ethical Issues

Besides the connection with the euthanasia movement mentioned above, there are three major ethical reasons given for not writing AHCDs. None of these reasons is insurmountable.

First, many question whether instructions in an advance directive can be truly informed. If a competent patient needs treatment, the doctor explains the options to her with accompanying risks and benefits and she can make her own decision. This is called informed choice or informed consent. How does one make decisions, however, if one does not know what he or she is going to face? If a patient has a massive stroke, will the decisions about treatment change as the daily prognosis changes? How does one anticipate the nuances of complex medical situations? For example, on the first day after a stroke, doctors often do not know whether the patient will improve or remain basically the same. By the seventh day, the prognosis is usually reasonably clear. What if an AHCD makes no distinction between the first and seventh days?

Second, and along the same lines, advance directives simply cannot anticipate all the conditions one might face. One of my favorite stories of an AHCD involved a doctor who tore up his directive after he reached page fifty and still hadn't covered issues around brain damage due to cancer! On the other hand, many AHCDs are so vague—requesting "no heroic measures" or "no extraordinary measures" or "I don't want to be kept alive with tubes"—that one has to wonder if some AHCDs are not simply an expression of a person's fears rather than well-thought-out directions for treatment.

Finally, AHCDs may tie the hands of health care providers. If a person writes, "I do not want to be on a ventilator," there is no distinction between being on a ventilator for the rest of one's life or for a few days to get over a crisis. A doctor reading this statement cannot presume that it means one or the other. So if read literally, no ventilator can be used and the patient may die quite unnecessarily.

Substitute Decision Makers

(Durable Powers of Attorney for Health Care, Proxies, Surrogate Decision Makers, Health Care Agents)

Most ethicists try to counter the above ethical issues by inviting patients to appoint a substitute decision maker (SDM) who has the right to make decisions for the noncompetent patient, based as far as possible on the patient's own wishes. Some ethicists think that no further written instructions are really needed. One writes a *proxy document* specifying who will be his/her SDM and then discusses what the decisions ought to be with this person. The SDM then "substitutes" for the patient who is unable to make or communicate decisions.

While such a model works for many people, it may not be enough. Sometimes, written instructions are needed to confirm that the SDM is following the patient's wishes and is not simply expressing his or her own desires under the pressure of a crisis. Terri Schiavo might have saved her family considerable difficulty by writing down her wishes. Sometimes, written instructions are needed to get all the family members to focus on whose decision counts, namely, the patient's. At other times, the law demands written instructions for the sake of certainty.

With all of this in mind, and in line with the thinking of many ethicists, a combination AHCD is recommended—one which appoints an SDM *and* provides written directions as far as possible. What follows is an attempt to guide the writing of such a document.

Preparing an Advance Health Care Directive

Preliminary Remarks

First, notice that modern-day ethicists and doctors are careful not to use the popular phrase "living will" with respect to AHCDs. Even though the term is often used, it is quite inaccurate. Wills are generally opened after one dies. An AHCD, on the other hand, is meant for use *before* bodily death. A "living will," therefore, is a contradiction in terms and will be avoided.

Second, it is important to recognize that every state and province has its own legislation about writing advance directives. Some demand the signature of a witness; some put a time limit on the document; some allow refusal of treatment resulting in death only under certain circumstances. Consequently, it is important to consult with a physician, lawyer, ethicist, or other knowledgeable person to ascertain what is legally permitted and required in one's particular state or province. In other words, the following procedures should serve as a guide for creating an AHCD, but careful attention should be paid to local and regional legal restrictions.

Appointing the Substitute Decision-Maker(s)

Undoubtedly, the single most important element in an AHCD is the choice of a substitute decision-maker. In choosing this person, be sure to choose somebody who knows you and knows your wishes. Generally, this will be a family member, but not necessarily. It may also be a good idea to add an alternate SDM to your document. If the first SDM is unavailable, then who would you want to decide in his/her place?

Some choose several SDMs. For example, a couple with three children wanted all three to be involved in the decision making. In such situations, I always advise that a specific method of choosing be given to this small group. Are they to come to a consensus? Would a majority decision be acceptable? Should the three discuss the situation, but have only one person who will communicate the decision(s) to the doctors? Occasionally, I have encountered statements like "any adult child can decide, but if there are any disagreements, then 'x' makes the final decision." One has to know his/her own family. If they are harmonious, then no problems should arise. If one member of the family tends to dominate, and not always reasonably, you may need to adjust your directions.

When you do choose your SDM(s), it is imperative to communicate this wish to your family so that they know a decision-maker is in place, should a crisis arise. Some family members are surprised when another family member suddenly produces a document and claims the right to decide. It is not uncommon for a son or daughter to suddenly show up from afar and attempt to "take over" the decisions for a parent. A written document does not allow this to happen. (On the other hand, if there is no SDM document, local legislation determines who makes the decisions—and sometimes that is the oldest child, even if he or she lives time-zones away and has hardly spoken to the parent for years.)

Also, for the benefit of all involved, it would be important to sort out as many family issues as possible *before* there is a crisis. Family disagreements at the bedside can be particularly distressing for caregivers as well as family members.

Once again, and finally, it is very important to check the legislation in your state or province. To write a document specifying your SDM may be very simple—a written or typed page, signed and dated—or there may be other specifics needed, such as a witness or a notary public. Occasionally, one must make use of a lawyer. Above all, be sure that the document is legally acceptable.

The Essential Components of an Advance Health Care Directive

Many people today opt only to write a proxy document, that is, they simply appoint a substitute decision maker who will look after treatment decisions during times of noncompetency. Others seek to give such SDMs more direction and choose to write some instructions. This may help the SDM to stand firm in the face of family opposition. It also might help the SDM to be sure about the person's wishes. And even if you do not write an AHCD, the following guidelines should help you to discuss most of the relevant issues with your SDM.

After appointing and clarifying the duties of your SDM, there are three essential things that need to go into a written advance health care directive.

First, if you are dying (and unable to make your own decisions), ask for palliative or hospice care, which is treatment appropriate for the dying. Such care helps to avoid overtreating and dragging out the dying process. At the same time, it avoids undertreating where the patient is left to unnecessarily endure excessive pain or physical distress. The patient's family or SDM(s) can work with the palliative/hospice team members to provide appropriate care for the dying person. Treatments will be proposed only as needed, their possible benefits and side effects will be discussed, and choices for the comfort of the patient will be respected.

Second, it is important to make a statement about your most fundamental beliefs. Hence, a Catholic might state something like, "I wish to be treated in accord with sound Catholic medical-moral principles." This would mean, for example, that extraordinary means of treatment can be foregone by the dying patient if such treatment would only prolong the dying process, be too painful or too burdensome, or have little chance of success. More and more, I also see this second statement to be a protection for Catholics whose respect for life, even when a person is close to death, is not always shared by some hospital personnel.

Third, it is helpful to put a "safety valve" statement in one's AHCD. "If you do not know what my condition is, please treat me until you do know; then follow my wishes—make me better if you can, or allow me to die according to my instructions (which my SDM knows or my AHCD expresses)." Such a sentence helps ensure that you are given every chance, especially in an emergency or critical situation. It demands treatment in the face of uncertainty. So, for example, an unconscious person might require dialysis in order to survive. The doctor is uncertain about the patient's future and is not sure about dialysis. However, by dialyzing a patient one may gain enough time for the rest of the body to begin to heal. On the other hand, if it is later determined that the patient is dying and nothing will stop the process, then he/she has not been harmed by the dialysis but the family/SDM is now more certain about the patient's condition. Accordingly, decisions can be made with more accuracy.

Specific Issues to Consider

There are a number of specific issues that one should think about concerning end-of-life choices. You may not face any of these issues, but if your family or SDM must make a decision, then your expressed wishes with regard to these situations are vital.

Some people do not specify anything about these situations because they fear a too-literal interpretation. Others feel that the circumstances can vary so much that they simply want their SDM to evaluate the ongoing situation and make decisions accordingly. Again, however, to have at least discussed these issues—even if one is not entirely sure what one might want—can be very valuable for those who need to make decisions based upon one's wishes. The 1979 case of Brother Fox (an eighty-three-year-old Christian Brother who fell into total unconsciousness after a routine hernia operation and heart attack during surgery) was settled to a great extent, not because he had written any instructions, but because he had often talked with his fellow Christian Brothers and his students, by making it clear that he would not want to be kept alive in an irreversibly unconscious state by the use of a ventilator.

What are your wishes concerning the following treatment options?

The use of a ventilator. Ventilators will breathe for the person unable to do so. They pump air into and out of the lungs. One may be unconscious, or paralyzed, or too weak to breathe on one's own. A ventilator can be a lifesaver.

However, ventilators can keep a dying person breathing, even when nothing else can be done to restore the person to health. Ventilators are sometimes used for an extended period of time (sometimes many years) for those who have sustained spinal cord injuries resulting in paralysis or who have suffered from diseases such as Guillain-Barré Syndrome. The competent patient can make a decision about continuing or stopping such treatment (depending upon its burden, and so forth. See, for example, the case of Nancy B in Canada, 1992).

What happens, though, when you are unable to make your own decisions? Would you want to be kept alive on a ventilator if you would never regain consciousness? If you would regain only minimal awareness? If you were dying from a serious illness and this was simply prolonging the dying process?

Recall, too, what was said above about the "safety valve" clause. If the ventilator is needed and your prognosis is uncertain, it is assumed that the ventilator will be used until a clearer prognosis is possible.

Cardio-pulmonary resuscitation (CPR). Whether through chest compressions or the use of defibrillators (which attempt to shock the heart back into action), CPR is often seen as a miracle intervention. Sometimes it is! Nonetheless, the success rate for CPR depends on many factors—elapsed time since heart stoppage, physical condition, illnesses, type of heart failure, and the like. Its success rate may be as high as 35 percent (in a hospital with staff and equipment) but the rate approaches less than 1 percent when dealing with the frail elderly in a nursing home. The older and more frail one is, and the more medical problems one has, the less chance of success.

When the heart stops irreversibly, the patient dies. Many people may not be ready to die—which is why CPR is automatically initiated in hospitals, unless the patient has expressly refused—but death cannot be postponed forever. Most people in palliative or hospice care, for example, choose not to have CPR (except under very special circumstances, like when a loved one from out of town is due to arrive shortly. But, of course, there is no guarantee that CPR will restore heart function). Such refusals of CPR are often called a DNR (Do Not Resuscitate, or Do Not Attempt Resuscitation) or a No Code (which means that the hospital staff will not call the code that initiates resuscitative interventions). Because CPR has often been used indiscriminately in hospitals, even at the end of life when death is inevitable, it is now more common to ask patients if they would be willing to forego any attempt at CPR.

In your AHCD, at what point would you be willing to authorize foregoing CPR? Know, too, that as a treatment intervention, not only does CPR have a low success rate, but sometimes, when it does succeed, it is at the cost of broken ribs, crushed chest cavities and bruised organs, or severe brain damage from lack of oxygen.

Surgery or aggressive interventions. Imagine yourself at the end of life, no longer able to make your own decisions because of an inability to think clearly or you are in some state of unconsciousness. What would you want your SDM to say to your doctors about aggressive treatments like surgery or chemotherapy? In such situations, you might write something such as "I would only accept surgery or aggressive medical interventions if they can make me better—including an ability to make my own decisions, even in a limited way—or if they will provide me with necessary pain control." Without such a statement, an aggressive doctor or surgeon might attempt to do something which *may* alleviate or correct one problem but which cannot cure you or stop the dying process.

It is not uncommon to include here even such seemingly "ordinary" treatments as the use of antibiotics. These wonder drugs can cure most infections. However, it can be unethical, for example, to try to cure pneumonia for a patient with end-stage lung cancer?

This may sound strange, but it can be considered ethical to die of pneumonia in this case rather than simply waiting for the cancer to run its course.

Feeding tubes. At present, there are three ways of nourishing or hydrating people who are unable to take food and water orally. First, doctors may order feeding tubes, either a naso-gastric tube (inserted through the nostril, down the throat, and into the stomach) or an enteral tube (which is surgically inserted directly into the stomach or into the small intestine). These methods provide nourishment without chewing and swallowing.

Second, a parenteral tube may be used, though usually only for a short term. It goes directly into a vein to supply nutrition and the stomach and intestine are bypassed.

Third, there are times when only hypodermoclysis is used. A needle is placed under the skin and water is trickled into the body to prevent dehydration problems. This is generally used when one cannot swallow and one's digestive system has failed. At times it is employed to help those suffering from cancer to remain hydrated.

Each of these treatments may be used with dying patients. Palliative/hospice caregivers are very careful, however, about recommending them. Contrary to what one might think, using any of these forms of nutrition and hydration might actually increase suffering for the dying. In a person whose digestive system is not working well or at all, for example, medically administered nutrition and hydration may cause bloating or other problems such as putting pressure on the heart or filling the lungs. This is one of the reasons why involving palliative care or hospice personnel in end-of-life decision making is so important. They understand that just because a treatment is available, it might not be beneficial to the patient.

When making a decision about the use of feeding tubes (or any other treatment), either for oneself or another, it is important to consider the basic principle that the Catholic tradition offers to guide such decisions, namely, the principle of proportionate/disproportionate means. The patient or the patient's SDM must weigh the burdens and benefits of the treatment relative to the patient's medical condition. If the benefits outweigh the burdens, from the patient's perspective, then the treatment would be considered morally obligatory. But if the treatment offers little or no hope of benefit to the patient or if the burdens outweigh any benefits, the patient or the patient's SDM may forgo the treatment. The *Ethical and Religious Directives for Catholic Health Care Services* speak of a "presumption in favor" of providing medically administered nutrition and hydration, but only as long as they are of sufficient benefit to outweigh the burdens involved to the patient (58). The *Health Ethics Guide* of the Canadian Catholic Conference of Bishops does not speak of such a presumption (100). In any case, one should never remove a feeding tube in order to bring about one's own or another's death.

Recently, considerable controversy has arisen regarding the removal of feeding tubes in patients who are in a persistent vegetative state (PVS). The Terri Schiavo case brought this issue to the fore in a very dramatic way. Less dramatic, but still very significant, was a talk by John Paul II in March 2004 in which the pope seemed to say that feeding tubes are generally morally required for patients in a PVS. The pope's statements resulted in considerable debate among clinicians, theologians, and laypeople because it seemed to differ from a five-hundred-year tradition within Catholicism regarding the prolongation of life as well as previous Church teaching. We cannot here go into the controversy surrounding this issue (it is dealt with more extensively in chapter 6). One should note, however, that official Church teaching on end-of-life treatment permits one in good conscience to refuse any treatment which will only prolong the dying process, which is too burdensome for oneself or one's family or community (whether physically, psychologically, or even financially), which has little chance of success, or which results in too great of side effects.

For our purposes, it is important to note that the pope was speaking about a specific class of patients (patients in a PVS) and that he seemed to be referring to patients in a PVS who had not previously expressed their wishes. He did not comment on making one's wishes known to one's family or SDM. Thus, we must be ever more vigilant about expressing our desire for end-of-life care, particularly since some states, following Terri Schiavo's death, introduced (and some passed) legislation that would require feeding tubes in patients who have not explicitly made their wishes known.

Because of the pope's statements, some Catholics will feel bound in conscience to use a feeding tube. Others will feel free to refuse based on an assessment of burdens and benefits in their particular situation. Both positions are true to the Church's teaching as long as there is not an official change in that teaching. People need to follow their *informed* conscience on this issue and then communicate their wishes to family and SDM.

For Whom Should You Write Your AHCD?

Should you write your AHCD for your SDM or for the doctor who might treat you? Most legislation makes it mandatory for a doctor to follow your written wishes. However, documents can often be ambiguous and what you write may be interpreted very differently by your doctor. Nonetheless, some people want this kind of protection, sometimes because they do not have an SDM willing to take responsibility for such decisions.

However, it has been my experience that if you write the AHCD for your SDM, he or she can then interpret what you have written and make decisions based upon your known, even if poorly expressed, wishes. For example, imagine a situation where a son interprets his father's vague AHCD to "refuse a feeding tube" to mean:

"Refuse the feeding tube only when I am irreversibly unconscious and unable to make decisions." The father had written "No feeding tubes" which he also discussed with his son. He later had a disorienting stroke which required the use of a feeding tube until he had sufficiently recovered his ability to eat on his own. The unwritten wishes of the patient, as represented by the son, prevailed. However, the vague AHCD without an SDM might have been taken literally by the doctor.

Conclusion

Advance health care directives will not take away the emotional upheaval that comes with making end-of-life decisions for a loved one. Facing mortality plus all the uncertainties around treatment options at the end of life is difficult and challenging.

Nonetheless, AHCDs will help. And they could make an enormous difference for you and your family. They can help properly focus the decision making on your wishes, and they can draw the family together in these decisions. And though they may not solve or anticipate every conceivable scenario, their presence will help alleviate some of the burdens that accompany end-of-life decisions.

Questions for Discussion

1. What are some of the advantages and disadvantages of advance health care directives?
2. Do you have an advance health care directive? If not, why not?
3. Have you ever had experience with an advance health care directive? Was that experience positive or negative? Explain.
4. Is there anything about advance health care directives that concerns you? If so, what is that and why?

For Further Reading

Catholic Conference of Kentucky. "Kentucky's Advance Health Care Directives and Organ Donation: A Catholic Perspective." September 2005, www.ccky.org/publications.htm. This is a pastoral letter of the bishops of Kentucky and provides both an explanation of advance directives from a Catholic perspective and a sample form.

Devine, Richard. "Death and Dying." In *Good Care, Painful Choices: Medical Ethics for Ordinary People*. Mahwah, N.J.: Paulist Press, 2004, 3rd ed., 201–223.

Christie, Dolores. *Last Rights: A Catholic Perspective on End-of-life Care*. Lanham, Md.: Rowman & Littlefield, 2003, 43–82.

Kelly, David. "Advance Directives." In *Contemporary Catholic Health Care Ethics*. Washington, DC: Georgetown University Press, 2004, 170–78.

O'Keefe, Mark. "Planning Now for Tough Medical Choices in the Future," *CareNotes*. St. Meinrad, Ind.: Abbey Press.

www.stpaulshospital.org. This site contains a sample AHCD for Catholics developed by the ethics committee of St. Paul's Hospital in Saskatoon, Saskatchewan, Canada. Readers are welcome to make use of it and to adapt it to fit their own circumstances.

CHAPTER 6

Making Decisions about Medically Administered Nutrition and Hydration

Michael R. Panicola, PhD

W hen I was a child, my grandfather suddenly became very ill and was eventually diagnosed with a malignant brain tumor. At first, this man, who was the epitome of strength and perseverance, fought hard against the disease. This included undergoing brain surgery, chemotherapy, and radiation. For a while, medicine's efforts and my grandfather's will to survive seemed to be winning out. However, it wasn't long before the disease regained the upper hand and my grandfather was forced to face the limits of medicine and his own existence.

I remember the day well. My grandmother picked me up after school, and we went to visit my grandfather at the hospital. After we had been there for a while, the doctor came into the room and informed him, in our presence, that the tumor was growing back and that he would need to undergo additional chemotherapy and possibly radiation. Though there seemed to be no choice in the matter, my grandfather, only a shadow of his former self in body, told the doctor that he had had enough and that he would not pursue any further treatment. The doctor seemed to accept my grandfather's decision rather easily. He quickly looked to my grandmother, who was visibly distraught, for her reaction. Before my grandmother could say anything, my grandfather took her hands into his own and, with quiet resolve, said: "Jean, I've done all I can do; now it's time we let go."

In many ways, this is an unremarkable story. Most of us have experienced the death of a loved one and the ups and downs that precede it. Yet there is one thing that stands out: my grandfather knew, with a level of certainty that is often hard to achieve, that he had done all *he* could to beat the disease, and that it made no sense to continue fighting with medical means given the inevitability of his own death. This is remarkable, especially when one considers the uncertainty that often characterizes treatment decisions at the end of life today. Unlike my grandfather, who knew that medicine had reached its limits and the time had come to let go, many of us nowadays have difficulty realizing and accepting this same fate. This is not because we are weaker persons than my grandfather nor have less faith than he did. Rather, it is because we are often ambivalent about just how far we can and should go to preserve our lives when confronted with a life-threatening illness. This ambivalence is not new; people of all ages have experienced it given the finality of death and the mystery that shrouds it. What makes it problematic today, though, is that medicine has tremendous capacity to stave off death, often times with mixed results.

Whereas in the not-too-distant past we died because of our illness, today we can often be kept alive by treating complications that arise with the numerous medical technologies at our disposal. Consequently, today's decisions at the end of life often revolve around whether to continue the breathing machine after a serious stroke, or to start the kidney machine to combat the effects of chronic liver disease, or to administer antibiotics to treat a serious infection, or to attempt resuscitation when the heart stops. With advances in medical technology, we must now face the harrowing task of determining, as my grandfather did, when it is time to let go because we have done all we can reasonably be expected to do to preserve our lives.

Even in the best of circumstances, these treatment decisions can be distressing and leave us filled with doubt as to the appropriateness of our choices. Perhaps the most troubling of all such decisions are those that involve feeding tubes or, what clinicians refer to as medically administered nutrition and hydration (MANH). Sometimes, because of an illness or injury, we lose the capacity to swallow and as a result must receive nutrients and fluids medically through an intravenous (or IV) line, or through a tube inserted into our nose (naso-gastric or NG), or surgically placed into our digestive tract (gastrostomy). Although feeding tube decisions are driven by the same moral considerations as other medical technologies, they tend to be much more emotionally challenging given the symbolic value we place on food and fluids, the images of starvation that often arise when we think of a person not eating, and the fact that they are often being made for individuals no longer able to make decisions for themselves.

Such decisions, while never easy, have become increasingly complex in recent years due largely to the controversy caused by highly publicized cases involving the removal of MANH from patients in what is called a persistent vegetative (or unconscious) state (PVS), especially the Terri Schiavo case (the Florida woman who was in a PVS for over fifteen years and died on March 31, 2005, after her feeding tube was removed two weeks earlier). Numerous courts, politicians, heath care professionals, theologians, ethicists, and ordinary citizens weighed in on the Schiavo case with conflicting positions and arguments, often on national newscasts and in local and major newspapers. For Catholics, the Schiavo case raised particular concerns and caused much confusion as some, including priests and high-ranking Church officials, described the removal of the feeding tube as "murder by starvation." To complicate matters, the late Pope John Paul II weighed in on the issue of nutrition and hydration prior to his own death by giving an address (or allocution) to a group of conference participants in March 2004. Far from clearing up the confusion, the papal allocution only added to it and left Catholics wondering where the Church stands on the use of MANH.

In what follows, I will attempt to bring some clarity to the issue by explaining what is required of us morally as Catholics when it comes to decisions about preserving our lives with medical means, in particular, MANH. Because tradition is one of the pillars of Catholic teaching, I will begin with a brief description of the centuries-old Catholic tradition on the duty to preserve life and then highlight some recent challenges to the traditional viewpoint. I will then provide a succinct summary and analysis of the recent papal allocution. By way of conclusion, I will point out where we stand in terms of current Church teaching and outline several moral norms for decision making that embody this teaching.

The Catholic Tradition

Catholic theologians have been writing on this very issue for some five hundred years. Even though medicine was relatively powerless throughout most of this time, questions still arose as to what our moral responsibility is to preserve our lives with medical means, including food and fluids. What the traditional theologians said is not only interesting, but it provides the basis for current Church teaching. The tradition is long and complex, but I will summarize it by highlighting three critical features.

MAKING DECISIONS ABOUT NUTRITION & HYDRATION   113

Duty to Preserve Life

The bedrock for the traditional viewpoint is found in the basic Christian understanding of life and death. As Christians, we believe that human life is a great good that has been given to us freely out of love by God. It is through life on earth that we are able to enter more fully into communion with God by loving others as God loves us. For these reasons, we have a strong moral duty to protect and to preserve our lives. Yet this duty is not absolutely binding under all circumstances because our ultimate end lies *not in this life* but in eternal life with God. To hold otherwise would be a denial of a central Christian belief, namely, that Jesus conquered death, through which we rise to new life.

This balanced view of life and death is important, because it stakes a middle ground between two extreme views that often creep up in the debate over the use of MANH. On one side are those who claim or imply that we have complete authority over our lives and, as such, can decide to do with it what we will, even ending it if we so choose. This argument is cited most often in support of euthanasia and assisted suicide. On the other side are those who claim or imply that life is an absolute good and as such it must be preserved at all costs regardless of the condition of the person. This argument is equally problematic because it limits human choice and condemns us to being held hostage by technology. The Christian view holds neither stance as an absolute, recognizing, on the one hand, a duty to preserve life, but, on the other, the human limits of this duty.

Just what these limits are is a question that has been given considerable attention in the tradition. It has been widely accepted among Catholic theologians since the sixteenth century that one need only employ "ordinary" means of preserving life but not means that are deemed "extraordinary," by which is meant measures that either fail to offer a proportionate hope of benefit or impose an excessive burden or excessive expense on the family or community.

This distinction between ordinary and extraordinary means was first articulated explicitly in 1595 by Dominican theologian Domingo Bañez and it is still operative today, though now the terms *proportionate* and *disproportionate* are more often used.

The Relative Norm

The terminology shift that has occurred in recent years was necessary because the meaning of ordinary and extraordinary began to be seriously misunderstood as medicine became more advanced and certain means of preserving life became more common. As a consequence, the *moral question* regarding the effects of a particular means on the person was reduced to a *technical question* about the means itself. Thus, if a means, irrespective of the concrete circumstances of the person, were an ordinary medical procedure or therapy based on its cost, availability, ease of use, and so on, it was wrongly deemed ordinary in the moral sense of the term and hence morally obligatory. For the traditional theologians, however, no means of preserving life could be considered ordinary apart from an assessment of the benefits and burdens relative to the person's overall situation (physical, social, spiritual, financial, and so forth).

This is substantiated in the most comprehensive historical study of the topic, the 1958 doctoral dissertation of Archbishop Emeritus Daniel A. Cronin (Hartford, CT) entitled *The Moral Law in Regard to the Ordinary and Extraordinary Means of Conserving Life*. In his study, Archbishop Cronin reviewed the work of virtually every theologian who commented on the issue up to the time of his writing and had this to say about ordinary means:

> In summary, therefore, we may say that the notion of proportionate hope of success and benefit is an essential part of the nature of ordinary means. Without this hope of benefit, a means is hardly an ordinary means and therefore is

not obligatory. In determining the presence of this hope of success and benefit, one must consider not only the *nature of the particular remedy or means involved,* but also *the relative condition of the person* who is to use this means. *Then, and then only,* can the moral obligation of using such a means be properly determined (emphasis added).

This relative understanding of means is also seen in recent authoritative Church documents. For instance, in the 1980 *Declaration on Euthanasia,* issued by the Congregation for the Doctrine of the Faith (CDF), we read:

It will be possible to make a correct judgment as to the means by studying *the type of treatment* to be used, its *degree of complexity* or risk, *its cost* and the possibilities of using it, and comparing these elements with the *result* that can be expected, taking into account the *state of the sick person* and his or her *physical and moral resources* (see section IV, emphasis added).

Likewise, Pope John Paul II stated in his 1995 encyclical letter *Evangelium Vitae:*

Certainly there is a moral obligation to care for oneself and to allow oneself to be cared for, but this duty *must take account of concrete circumstances.* It needs to be determined whether the *means of treatment* available are objectively *proportionate to the prospects for improvement* (see number 65, emphasis added).

Nutrition and Hydration

For much of the history of the Church, traditional theologians did not have to contend with questions surrounding MANH. Feeding tubes were not available. Nevertheless, the traditional theologians did consider the moral obligation one has to preserve life with customary food and fluids. Given what was said above, it is not surprising that they held that even such common means could be forgone if they failed to provide a proportionate hope of benefit or imposed excessive burdens. The great Dominican theologian Francisco de Vitoria made this clear in the sixteenth century when he argued that

> if the depression of spirit is so low and there is present such consternation in the appetitive power that only with the greatest of effort and as though by means of a certain torture, can the sick man take food, right away that is reckoned a certain impossibility, and therefore he is excused, at least from mortal sin, especially where there is little hope of life or none at all.

De Vitoria's views were not unique among traditional theologians, as indicated by Archbishop Cronin:

> Even the older moralists teach that *such a purely ordinary and common means of conserving life as food, admits of relative inconvenience and difficulty.* Furthermore, they point out that this very common means, food, *sometimes can offer no proportionate hope of success* relative to a particular individual (emphasis added).

Nor were de Vitoria's views subsequently rejected by contemporary theologians, as evidenced by the large contingent of Catholic theologians who have written on the subject, espousing essentially the same view (for example, see Gerald Kelly, SJ; Benedict Ashley, OP; Kevin O'Rourke, OP; Richard McCormick, SJ; John Paris, SJ; Lisa Cahill; James Walter; Thomas Shannon; and Rev. Dennis Brodeur).

Recent Challenges to the Tradition

The Catholic tradition on the duty to preserve life has remained substantively the same from the sixteenth century through the present day. The wisdom of the tradition on questions of preserving life cannot be overstated nor has it gone unnoticed as its fundamental tenets have been incorporated into the legal and moral mind-set of the United States and other countries. Curiously, there have been some attempts recently to revise this tradition. Since the CDFs *Declaration on Euthanasia* in 1980, alternative viewpoints on the use of nutrition and hydration have appeared in several Church-related documents. While these documents challenge traditional thinking, it should be noted that they do not change Church teaching. They do not have the same theological weight as a declaration, an encyclical, or hundreds of years of theological reflection. Nonetheless, it is important to underscore the two significant ways in which these documents depart from the tradition because they serve as precursors to the papal allocution.

Nutrition and Hydration Always Obligatory

The first substantial departure from the tradition occurs in documents that classify nutrition and hydration, even artificially supplied, as care, basic care, or minimal measures for sustaining life, and then conclude that the provision of such care is always morally obligatory. For example, in its 1981 document, "Questions of Ethics Regarding the Fatally Ill and Dying," the Pontifical Council on Health Affairs stated:

There remains the strict obligation to apply under all circumstances those therapeutic measures which are called "minimal": that is, those which are normally and customarily used for the maintenance of life (alimentation, blood transfusions, injections, etc.). To interrupt these minimal measures would, in practice, be equivalent to wishing to put an end to the patient's life (2.4.4).

Similarly, the New Jersey Catholic Conference, in its 1987 statement, "Providing Food and Fluids to Severely Brain Damaged Patients," maintained that "nutrition and hydration, being *basic to human life,* are aspects of *normal care,* which are not excessively burdensome, that should *always be provided* to a patient" (emphasis added).

By classifying MANH as care that is always obligatory, these documents attempt to establish an absolute norm for its use. This is a major departure from the thought of traditional theologians, who, as we have seen, resisted such a temptation because they believed that relative factors (or concrete circumstances) needed to be taken into account before declaring any means—including nutrition and hydration—ordinary in the moral sense. Reflecting on how the traditional theologians viewed the matter of an absolute norm, Archbishop Cronin had this to say:

It is hardly possible *to establish categorically* that a particular means will always offer proportionate benefit under all circumstances and to all people. In other words, it is *difficult to establish an absolute norm* when determining the required hope of success and benefit in *any procedure* designed to conserve life (emphasis added).

For the traditional theologians, the decisive moral question was not how basic a particular means was to life or how common or easily available it was. Rather, it was whether the means offered a proportionate hope of benefit without imposing excessive burdens relative to the person's overall situation.

Meaning of "Benefit" Severely Restricted

The second substantial departure from the tradition occurs in documents that restrict the notion of benefit simply to sustaining life. For example, in "Nutrition and Hydration: Moral and Pastoral Reflections," the U.S. Bishops' Pro-Life Committee commented in 1992 that "such measures [nutrition and hydration] must not be withdrawn in order to cause death, but they may be withdrawn if they offer no reasonable hope of *sustaining life* or pose excessive risks or burdens" (emphasis added).

In a major shift, the Pro-Life Committee replaced the traditional language of "proportionate hope of benefit" with "reasonable hope of sustaining life." This limited physical understanding of benefit is not the way traditional theologians understood it. The simple fact that a means was capable of sustaining life did not necessarily mean that it provided a proportionate hope of benefit to the person. De Vitoria argued this point when he stated that

one is not held to lengthen his life, because he is not held to use always the most delicate foods, that is, hens and chickens, even though he has the ability and the doctors say that if he eats in such a manner, *he will live 20 years more*; and even if he knew this for certain, he would not be obliged (emphasis added).

Admittedly, the notion of "benefit" is hard to define because of the relative factors involved. I know no better way to convey its

meaning than by sharing a personal story. My mother was diagnosed with ovarian cancer. When it was finally discovered, the cancer had already metastasized. The doctors were not optimistic about
her prospects, but told her that with investigational chemotherapy
they might be able to buy her some time, perhaps as much as a year.
If sustaining life were the sole benefit my mom was considering, she
would have jumped at the chance. However, she debated whether to
undergo chemotherapy at all. In talking with the doctors about treatment, she wanted to know: how much pain she would experience;
whether her insurance covered the costs; how her relationships with
me and other loved ones would be affected; how much time she
would have to spend in the hospital; and whether she would be physically capable of working and pursuing her life's passion of painting.

This story provides insight into what the traditional theologians
meant by "proportionate hope of benefit." My mom knew intuitively
what the tradition has taught for centuries, namely, that sustaining
life is a benefit to the extent that it enables one to pursue the goals
of life that transcend physical life itself, at least at a minimal level,
without experiencing excessive burdens. This may sound complicated. However, all it really means is that we do not live life simply
so that our vital physiological functions can be maintained, but
rather so that we can pursue moral, spiritual, intellectual, and social goals that make up the sum and substance of human life. For
my mom, and I suspect most of us, these goals included pursuing
personal interests, engaging loved ones, deepening her relationship
with God, and contributing to society. In questioning the doctors,
what my mom really wanted to know was whether treatment would
give her the best chance of pursuing these goals, or whether she
would be profoundly frustrated in her pursuit of them in the mere
effort to survive. After receiving some assurances of the former, she
decided for treatment because she believed that it would provide,
on balance, more benefits than burdens. Importantly, though, it

wasn't length of life that was the primary consideration, but the type of life she would live in the time that she had left. This is what the traditional theologians had in mind when they talked about benefit and why de Vitoria could say that a person is not always obligated to use a certain means when it can sustain life, even for twenty years.

The Papal Allocution

What has been said to this point provides the background for understanding the papal allocution, delivered at an international conference held in Vatican City. The conference, "Life Sustaining Treatments and Vegetative State: Scientific Advances and Ethical Dilemmas," focused on ethical issues that arise in the care of patients in a PVS, particularly the issue of forgoing MANH. Before the close of the conference, on March 20, 2004, Pope John Paul II addressed the participants.

One part of the pope's address is particularly important for our purposes. However, before discussing it, I would like to provide a sketch of the contents of the allocution. In his comments, the pope emphasized: that patients in a PVS have an inherent dignity that is not lost because of their illness; that caregivers, families, and society have a duty to care for and protect these patients; that caregivers should be careful in diagnosing this condition because there are reports of misdiagnosis; that appropriate rehabilitative services should be provided to these patients because their condition is not necessarily helpless; that the term *vegetative* is not appropriate because it suggests these patients are less valuable than other persons; and that we can never remove treatment from these patients with the intention of killing them (doing so would be euthanasia by omission).

If this were all the pope said, we probably would not be talking about the allocution today. However, the pope made additional state-

ments that delighted some and shocked others, the most notewor-
thy of which include the following:

> The sick person in a vegetative state, awaiting recovery or a
> natural end, still has the right to basic health care (nutri-
> tion, hydration, cleanliness, warmth, etc.), and to the pre-
> vention of complications related to his confinement to bed.
> …I should like particularly to underline how the adminis-
> tration of water and food, even when provided by artificial
> means, always represents a *natural means* of preserving life,
> not a medical act. Its use, furthermore, should be consid-
> ered, in principle, *ordinary* and *proportionate,* and as such
> morally obligatory, insofar as and until it is seen to have
> attained its proper finality, which in the present case con-
> sists in providing nourishment to the patient and allevia-
> tion of his suffering (number 4, original emphasis).

Some welcomed these comments as a tightening of Catholic
principles on the moral duty to preserve life with MANH. Others
found these comments to be a significant departure from the tradition and a clear acceptance of recent challenges to it. What did the
pope actually mean by this statement?

Before analyzing the pope's comments, it is important to note
that while a papal allocution should be considered ordinary papal
teaching, allocutions are low-ranking teachings that, as Richard
McBrien describes in the *Encyclopedia of Catholicism,* do not ordinarily "contain material of legislative import" but merely express
"the pope's thoughts or opinions" on a given topic. In other words,
allocutions are not typically used to change Church teaching, especially teaching that is rooted in centuries of tradition. Still, we must
give an allocution respectful consideration.

Turning to the passage just quoted, the pope makes a general comment about nutrition and hydration and applies it specifically to patients in a PVS. The general comment indicates that nutrition and hydration, including MANH, should be considered, "in principle, ordinary and proportionate, and as such morally obligatory, insofar as and until it is seen to have attained its proper finality." Recalling the traditional theologians' views, this is a departure from their thought in that it elevates MANH to a special class of means of preserving life that must be considered ordinary, in principle, apart from concrete circumstances. Prior to the pope's allocution, there are no other examples of this way of thinking about means. At most we have an "in principle" obligation to preserve our lives, but not to use a certain means. If true of nutrition and hydration, why should it not be true of oxygen provided by a breathing machine? Importantly, though, the pope does not say that MANH is always ordinary and hence absolutely required. This he makes clear by saying that MANH is obligatory "insofar as and until it is seen to have attained its proper finality." Thus, in the pope's opinion, MANH is required morally insofar as it attains its proper finality.

What is its "proper finality"? The pope only provides an answer for patients in a PVS. For all others, he leaves it open-ended. This he does by saying "in the present case [by which he means PVS] consists in providing nourishment to the patient and alleviation of his suffering." Thus, nourishment and alleviation of suffering are the proper finality of MANH for patients in a PVS. If MANH is achieving these ends, then, in the pope's opinion, it is ordinary and hence morally obligatory. This may seem benign and the pope may have been hoping to protect vulnerable PVS patients from carelessness or malice. Nonetheless, it seems to be a departure from the tradition in that the pope's statement and not the PVS patient or the patient's family defines what the benefits and burdens are in light of the concrete and often changing circumstances.

Concluding Comments

So where does this leave us as Catholics? Like the documents that have recently challenged the tradition, though with somewhat more weight, the papal allocution does not change Catholic teaching on the duty to preserve life. It must be remembered that the allocution focused on a very specific and rare clinical condition, PVS, and many of the comments within it do not make good medical or moral sense for patients who more commonly are not able to eat or drink on their own because of illness or progressive disease (for example, end-stage cancer and advanced dementia). For these patients, evidence exists and experience shows that, in many instances, MANH does not confer any real benefit and can even impose undue and excessive burdens. Not starting or removing MANH in such instances would not be a form of euthanasia, but instead be recognition of the limits of medicine and of human existence.

So, in answer to the question above, we must turn to the long-standing tradition of the Church. As it was in the past, Catholic teaching still holds that: human life is a great good; we have a strong moral obligation to preserve life; there are limits to this obligation when it comes to using medical means, including MANH; and these limits are determined by considering the benefits and burdens of the means relative to the person's overall situation. The substance of these traditional norms is reflected in three of the *Ethical and Religious Directives for Catholic Health Care Services*. These directives provide a helpful summary of current Church teaching on the matter and also serve as a useful guide for decision making.

Directive 56: A person has a moral obligation to use ordinary or proportionate means of preserving his or her life. Proportionate means are those that in the judgment of the patient offer a reasonable hope of benefit and do not entail an excessive burden or impose excessive expense on the family or the community.

Directive 57: A person may forgo extraordinary or disproportionate means of preserving life. Disproportionate means are those that in the patient's judgment do not offer a reasonable hope of benefit or entail an excessive burden, or impose an excessive expense on the family or the community.

Directive 58: There should be a presumption in favor of providing nutrition and hydration to all patients, including patients who require medically assisted nutrition and hydration, as long as this is of sufficient benefit to outweigh the burdens involved to the patient.

Questions for Discussion

1. If you had to make a decision about withholding or withdrawing a feeding tube for yourself or a loved one, what would you consider?
2. What do you think you might consider to be the benefits and burdens in a decision about withholding or withdrawing a feeding tube for yourself?
3. Would you want a feeding tube if you were dying or you were permanently unconscious? Explain.
4. Given the Catholic emphasis on the duty to preserve life, how might you respond to someone who says that withdrawing a feeding tube is nothing short of euthanasia?

For Further Reading

Cahill, Lisa Sowle. "Catholicism, Death and Modern Medicine." *America* (25 April 2005):14–17.

Congregation for the Doctrine of the Faith. "Declaration on Euthanasia." *Origins* 10 (August 14, 1980): 154–57.

Hamel, Ronald and Michael Panicola. "Must We Preserve Life?" *America* (April 19–26, 2004): 6–13.

Pope John Paul II, "Care for Patients in a 'Permanent' Vegetative State," *Origins* 33 (April 8, 2004): 737, 739–40.

McCormick, Richard. "Nutrition-Hydration: The New Euthanasia?" In *Critical Calling.* Washington, DC: Georgetown University Press, 1989: 369–88.

Myers, Archbishop John. "End-of-life Decisions: Ethical Principles." *Origins* 35 (September 22, 2005): 248–53.

Panicola, Michael R. "Catholic Teaching on Prolonging Life." *Hastings Center Report* 31 (November–December, 2001): 14–25.

Sheehan, Myles N. "Feeding Tubes: Sorting Out the Issues." *Health Progress* 82 (November–December, 2001): 22–27.

Glossary

Advance Health Care Directive (AHCD) A document that informs others of (1) one's wishes regarding medical treatment in the event one is unable to make decisions for oneself or is unable to communicate those wishes, or (2) the individual that one has chosen to make decisions for oneself, i.e., one's surrogate decision maker, or (3) both one's wishes and one's surrogate decision maker. The first type of document is often referred to as a "living will" or an "instructional directive" while the second is called a "durable power of attorney for health care" or a "proxy directive." The third type of document is a combination of both.

Allowing to Die In the Catholic tradition, allowing to die involves the withholding or withdrawing of life-sustaining treatment that is judged by the patient or the patient's family or surrogate to be excessively burdensome and/or of little or no benefit. It involves a decision to no longer prevent the underlying disease process or pathology to run its course.

Amniocentesis A form of prenatal diagnosis that collects fetal cells from the amniotic fluid to test whether the fetus is a carrier of or is affected with a genetic condition. It involves inserting a needle through the mother's abdominal wall into the uterine cavity and is generally performed between the fifteenth and twentieth weeks of pregnancy.

Autonomy A central principle, especially in secular medical ethics. It refers to an individual's right to make decisions for oneself on the basis of one's freely chosen values, goals, life plan, and so on.

"Best Interests" Standard The standard employed to make treatment decisions when a person's wishes or preferences are not known or are unclear. The substitute decision maker seeks to choose that course of action that he or she believes will promote the "best interests" or welfare of the patient.

Carrier   A person who has a recessive mutated gene along with a normal copy of the same gene. Carriers do not usually develop the disease caused by the mutation, but they can pass the mutated gene to their children. If two carriers with the same mutated gene reproduce, each child has a 25 percent probability of acquiring the disease, a 50 percent probability of being a carrier, and a 25 percent chance of being unaffected (i.e., having the normal gene).

Chromosome   Structures found in the nucleus of a cell that contain the genes. Chromosomes come in pairs. A normal human cell contains forty-six chromosomes, twenty-two pair of autosomes (non-sex determining chromosomes) and two sex chromosomes (XX or XY).

Cloning   Cloning involves taking a human egg, removing the nucleus, and replacing that nucleus with the nucleus of an ordinary body cell. The single cell is stimulated to divide. Each cell resulting from the division is genetically identical to the body cell and to the individual from whom it was taken.

Complicity   Refers to some form of involvement in the evildoing of others.

Consistent Ethic of Life   A moral perspective proposed by the late Joseph Cardinal Bernardin in 1983 that argues for a relationship among all issues that threaten human life and human dignity, that is, abortion and euthanasia, for example, as well as poverty and racism. His proposal is also sometimes referred to as the "seamless garment."

Competency   In health care, competency refers to one's ability to make treatment decisions or one's decision making capacity. It involves the ability to understand relevant information including treatment options, to appreciate the significance of one's medical condition and the major risks and benefits of the treatment options, to reason about treatment options in relation to one's values and preferences, and to communicate a choice. Generally, it is limited to the ability to make a particular decision.

CPR   A shorthand for cardiopulmonary resuscitation which involves various methods for reversing cardiac or respiratory arrest. These methods include chest compressions, assisted ventilation, defibrillation, and the use of drugs.

Cystic Fibrosis A common genetic disorder, especially in the Caucasian population. The disease causes thick mucous to accumulate affecting the lungs, pancreas, and digestive tract and shows a wide range of severity. Aggressive treatment has extended the lifespan of children with CF into their late twenties and even beyond.

Donation after Cardiac Death (DCD) The removal of organs from someone who is declared dead after the cessation of spontaneous heartbeat and respiration. This stands in contrast to the removal of organs from someone who is brain dead, but whose heartbeat and respiration are maintained by a ventilator and medications.

DNR Do-not-resuscitate. A medical order not to employ various measures to restore heartbeat and respiration after someone's heart has stopped beating.

Differentiation The process whereby early cells which are capable of becoming any cell begin to "specify," to become particular types of cells, for example, heart, lung, brain, and so forth.

Double Effect A basic principle in Catholic moral theology that helps guide decisions about performing actions that have two effects—one good and intended and the other bad and unintended. The principle holds that one may perform such actions if (1) the action is good or neutral in itself; (2) one intends the good effect and not the bad; (3) the good and bad effects occur together so that the evil effect does not become a means to the good effect, and (4) there is a proportionately serious reason for allowing the unintended bad effect to occur. A classic example is the removal of a cancerous uterus which both saves the mother's life, but also makes her sterile.

Durable Power of Attorney for Health Care A document in which one appoints someone to makes decisions for oneself should one become incapacitated. The person named is one's surrogate or proxy decision maker.

Encyclical A formal pastoral letter written by the pope on some doctrinal, moral, or disciplinary matter and which is addressed to the universal church.

Ethical and Religious Directives for Catholic Health Care Services   A brief document published by the United States Conference of Catholic Bishops that provides moral guidance on various aspects of health care delivery to all those who are in some way associated with Catholic health care facilities, whether administrators, health care professionals and staff, or patients and their families.

Ethics   The study of the rightness and wrongness of human choice and actions and the goodness and badness of character, that is, the study of how we ought to behave and the kinds of persons and communities we ought to become. Some make a distinction between "morality" and "ethics" where morality refers to one's actual values, choices, and actions in daily living, while ethics is the theoretical and systematic study of morality. However, many today use the terms interchangeably.

Euthanasia   An action or an omission which directly and intentionally brings about a terminally ill person's death in order to relieve suffering.

Gene   A gene is an ordered sequence of nucleotides located in a particular position on a particular chromosome that encodes a specific functional product, such as a protein.

Genetic Counseling   An educational process that helps individuals, couples, or families to understand genetic information and issues that may have an impact on them.

Genetic Screening   Testing groups of individuals to determine whether a particular gene is present that could cause an inherited condition.

Genetic Testing   Examining a blood, body fluid, or tissue sample for biochemical, chromosomal, or genetic markers that indicate the presence or absence of genetic disease.

Health Care Ethics Guide   A publication of the Catholic Health Association of Canada with the approval of the Canadian Conference of Catholic Bishops that provides guidance to a variety of audiences in addressing a range of ethical issues in the health care arena.

Hemochromatosis   A genetic disorder of iron metabolism. Presence of the gene mutation may or may not lead to symptoms. When identified clinically, the disorder can be effectively treated through bloodletting.

Huntington's Disease   An adult-onset disease characterized by progressive mental and physical deterioration, eventually ending in death.

Informed Consent A process whereby an individual is provided adequate information about a treatment option, its risks and benefits, alternatives and their risks and benefits, is able to understand and appreciate the significance of the information, and makes an uncoerced choice about a particular option. It is an expression of respect for human dignity and patient autonomy and is the usual vehicle for a patient's expression of his or her treatment preferences. Informed consent is central to the health professional-patient relationship. Generally, requires conversation and is not adequately achieved by the provision and signing of a form.

In Vitro Fertilization The union of sperm and egg and subsequent cell division in a laboratory dish. Generally, several eggs are fertilized at one time and several embryos are implanted. Any remaining embryos are either frozen or discarded. The Church prohibits in vitro fertilization because it involves the creation of new life apart of an act of sexual intercourse between spouses and because of the deliberate destruction of embryos.

Living Will A document that expresses one's preferences about medical treatment in the event that one is not able to make decisions for oneself. Also called an "instruction directive."

Magisterium The teaching role and authority of the Catholic Church as residing in the pope and the bishops.

Mutation A change in the number, arrangement, or molecular sequence of a gene that can be inherited.

Noncompetent Lacking the ability to make decisions for oneself.

Physician Assisted Suicide The assistance of a physician in bringing about one's own death when one is terminal.

Preimplantation Genetic Diagnosis The use of in vitro fertilization to enable genetic diagnosis of the embryo at two to four days after fertilization and before implantation. Generally, only embryos free of a genetic mutation are implanted. The others are usually discarded.

Prenatal Diagnosis Diagnostic procedures performed to identify fetal defects during pregnancy which include ultrasound, amniocentesis (performed at fifteen to twenty weeks), chorionic villus sampling (between ten and thirteen weeks), and maternal serum screening (noninvasive).

Proxy Decision Maker   One who "stands in" for another person who is not capable of making his or her own decisions. The proxy's decision as much as possible should reflect the one that he or she knows or believes the patient would have made if capable. If this is unknown, then the proxy should decide what is in the patient's best interests. The proxy's decision normally should be followed provided it is made in good faith and is consistent with church teaching.

Reproductive Cloning   Cloning that is employed to create a human being with the intention of bringing it to term.

Resuscitation   Restarting the heart of someone whose heart has stopped beating and who has stopped breathing. Reversal of cardiac or respiratory arrest.

Stewardship   The responsibility that human beings have to care for the gift of their lives, their bodies, and all of creation.

Therapeutic Cloning   The use of cloning to create human embryos for research purposes or to extract embryonic stem cells.

Utilitarianism   A perspective that judges something on the basis of its utility or usefulness.

Index